FOODS LISTS FOR KIDNEY DISEASE 2024

INCLUDES 2,000 KIDNEY FRIENDLY FOODS LIST WITH LOW SODIUM, LOW POTASSIUM, LOW PHOSPHORUS CONTENTS + 30 MEAL PLANS FOR STAGES 2, 3, 4, & 50 KIDNEY FRIENDLY RECIPES

JULIA MEADOWS

ABOUT THE AUTHOR

Julia Meadows is a health professional and wellness expert, specialising in nutrition she has delivered life-changing transformations for her readers.

She's residing with her family; husband, 2 boys and a girl, 2 cats and dog in the beautiful countryside of Sussex, just outside of London, England.

As a master health & wellness expert Julia teaches clients on consciousness, mindful living, nutrition, health care and diet, and good food for the mind, body and soul. Through our teaching Julia has helped clients worldwide gain a better advantage and help develop themselves and achieve more from what they desire.

She's in the changing lives business.

TAKE YOUR LIFESTYLE JOURNEY TO THE NEXT LEVEL!

http://www.facebook.com/groups/glycemic/

In our exclusive Diabetic and Low-Glycemic Information group, you'll connect with like-minded individuals who are embarking on the same wellness journey. It's a space where you can share your personal experiences, triumphs, and challenges, and also learn from others' experiences.

Plus, it's not just a community — it's a vast resource. You'll gain access to insider tips, recipe ideas, motivational stories, and expert advice from experienced like-mind followers. To become part of our thriving Facebook group, simply search 'Diabetes & Low Glycemic Nutrition Information' on Facebook, and hit 'Join'. We can't wait to welcome you to our community and watch you thrive on your Healthy Life-style journey!"

GET YOUR 7 BONUSES:

RENAL DIET & DASH DIET 2024 BOOKS
DIABETES: GUIDE AND EXERCISES EBOOKS
TRACKERS
AUDIOBOOKS
VIDEO COURSE

TOTAL REALISTIC VALUE OF ALL FREE BONUSES ABOVE:
$350 FOR FREE!

SCAN THE QR CODE!

BONUS 1 AND 2/7: DASH DIET AND RENAL DIET 2024 BOOKS!

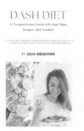

This comprehensive guide delivers a strategy for managing CKD and Hypertension. It provides an array of meal plans and low-sodium recipes with printable templates for 7-day food diary, 5-weeks meal planner, and 30-days of exercise log.

Value: $100- for **FREE!**
QR Code Below

BONUS 3 and 4/7- 2 EBOOKS

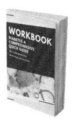
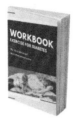

Diabetes A
Comprehensive
Quick Guide
Book 1
Best Selling Amazon Author

Exercise For
Diabetes
Book 2
Best Selling Amazon Author

- 1. Diabetes: A Comprehensive Guide
- 2. Exercise for Diabetes Workouts & Meal Plans

This essential workbook serves as a comprehensive tool for improved wellness.

Value: $50- for **Free!**
QR Code Below

BONUS 5/7- TRACKERS & WORKBOOKS

Trackers,
Planners & Cheat
Sheets

- 1. Sodium Tracker
- 2. Blood Sugar Tracker
- 3. Cholesterol Tracker

This is a set of comprehensive tools designed to help you monitor and track your health metrics.

Value: $100- for **Free!**
QR Code Below

BONUS 6/7- AUDIOBOOKS

- CHINESE HERBS
- HOW TO BOOST YOUR METABOLISM
- HOW TO LOSE 10 POUNDS NATURALLY
- NATURAL REMEDIES
- HEALTHY WEIGHT LOSS

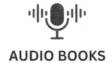

AUDIO BOOKS

Value: $60- Cost **Free!**

QR Code Below

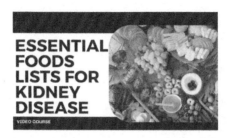

This comprehensive guide offers expert advice and practical tips on identifying low-sodium foods, understanding labels, and making healthier grocery choices to reduce sodium intake and enhance overall health.

Value: $60- Cost **Free!**
QR Code Below

GET YOUR 7 BONUSES:

RENAL DIET & DASH DIET 2024 BOOKS
DIABETES: GUIDE AND EXERCISES EBOOKS
TRACKERS
AUDIOBOOKS
VIDEO COURSE

TOTAL REALISTIC VALUE OF ALL FREE BONUSES ABOVE:
$350 FOR FREE!

SCAN THE QR CODE!

MASTERSHIP BOOKS

UK | USA | Canada | Ireland | Australia
India | New Zealand | South Africa | China
Mastership Books is part of the United Arts Publishing House group
of companies based in London, England, UK.
First published by Mastership Books (London, UK), 2023
Text Copyright © United Arts Publishing
Cover design by Rich © United Arts Publishing (UK)
Text and internal design by Rich © United Arts Publishing (UK)
Image credits reserved.
Color separation by Spitting Image Design Studio
Printed and bound in Great Britain
National Publications Association of Britain
London, England, United Kingdom.
Paper design UAP
A723.5
Title: Foods Lists For Kidney Disease 2024
Design, Bound & Printed:
London, England,
Great Britain.

FREE BOOK CLUB:

Email me:
juliameadowsauthor@gmail.com

CONTENTS

INTRODUCTION

Proper nutrition plays a vital and indispensable role in the effective management of kidney disease, as it can significantly slow down the progression of this condition. When the kidneys are not functioning optimally, making specific dietary modifications becomes crucial to minimize waste products and fluid accumulation in the bloodstream. Moreover, these modifications can effectively alleviate symptoms associated with kidney disease, such as swelling, fatigue, and poor appetite. By following a well-balanced diet, individuals can not only protect their kidneys from further damage but also regulate blood pressure and blood sugar levels, leading to an overall improvement in their health and well-being. Therefore, emphasizing the importance of maintaining a nutritious diet is essential for individuals with kidney disease.

This book aims to provide readers with a comprehensive guide on the essential foods beneficial for kidney disease. It aims to empower those dealing with kidney disease and their caregivers with knowledge about dietary modifications that can aid in managing the condition. The book is structured into sections focusing on various food groups, explaining their impact on kidney health, and providing lists of kidney-friendly foods. In addition, each section contains practical tips and recipes to incorporate these foods into daily meals. Ultimately, this book is a valuable resource for anyone keen to understand the importance of diet in kidney disease management.

1

KIDNEY FUNCTIONS AND CHRONIC KIDNEY DISEASE (CKD)

This chapter provides a brief overview of the functions of the kidneys and how they are affected by chronic kidney disease (CKD). The kidneys play a critical role in filtering waste products, excess fluids, and toxins from the blood. They also help regulate blood pressure, produce red blood cell production hormones, and maintain mineral balance.

1.1. Understanding Kidney Functions

Our bodies' overall health greatly depends on the proper functioning of our kidneys, which are two bean-shaped organs in the lower back. They are the unsung heroes of our body, performing many tasks crucial for maintaining our health and well-being.

The kidneys act as the body's natural filtration system, processing around 200 quarts of blood daily to sift out about 2 quarts of waste products and extra water. This waste becomes urine, stored in the bladder before being expelled from the body. In addition, kidneys are responsible for maintaining a stable balance of salts, potassium, and acid in the body - elements that are essential for a range of bodily functions, encompassing nerve function to muscle contraction.

Furthermore, our kidneys regulate the levels of essential substances in our body, such as calcium and phosphate. They produce a hormone called calcitriol, pivotal in absorbing calcium and phosphate from our food, thereby maintaining strong bones and teeth.

Also, kidneys produce a hormone called erythropoietin that stimulates the bone marrow to make red blood cells. When the kidneys aren't functioning optimally, they make less erythropoietin, resulting in fewer red blood cells to carry oxygen. This condition is known as anemia, which can make a person feel tired and short of breath.

Understanding our kidneys' vital roles can enlighten us about maintaining our health and well-being. By incorporating kidney-friendly foods into our diet, as this book will guide you, we can significantly contribute to the overall health of our kidneys.

1.2. What is Chronic Kidney Disease?

Chronic Kidney Disease (CKD), as the name implies, is a long-term condition where the kidneys do not work as effectively as they should. It is characterized by the gradual loss of kidney function over time. This can range from mild dysfunction, often without noticeable symptoms, to severe kidney failure that requires dialysis or a kidney transplant. There are five stages of CKD, with stage 1 being the mildest and stage 5 (also referred to as End-Stage Renal Disease, or ESRD) being the most serious.

Unlike Acute Kidney Injury (AKI), which happens suddenly, often due to an injury or poisoning, CKD develops slowly, often over many years, and is usually caused by other long-term health conditions that damage the kidneys over time, such as diabetes and high blood pressure. While AKI may be reversible if detected and treated promptly, CKD is usually not reversible. Instead, treatments for CKD are focused on slowing down the progression of the disease.

In the early stages of CKD, there may be few signs or symptoms, and many people don't realize they have this condition. As CKD progresses, one might experience symptoms like fatigue, swelling in the legs, ankles, or feet, changes in urination patterns, and loss of appetite, among others. If left untreated, CKD can lead to complications like high blood pressure, anemia, weak bones, poor nutritional health, and nerve damage.

Understanding CKD and its progression is crucial as it enables timely interventions, significantly slowing the disease's progression and improving the quality of life for individuals with this condition. By making informed dietary choices, maintaining a healthy lifestyle, and following medical advice, we can manage CKD effectively and lead a fulfilling life.

1.3 Symptoms of Chronic Kidney Disease

Chronic Kidney Disease (CKD) may not present noticeable symptoms in its early stages, making it a somewhat silent disease. However, as kidney function declines, several symptoms may manifest, offering warning signs of the condition. These symptoms should never be ignored, as early detection and diagnosis can significantly slow CKD progression.

One of the first signs of CKD is changes in urination patterns. This can include an increase or decrease in frequency, blood in the urine, or the urine appearing foamy or bubbly. You might also experience difficulty while urinating or a persistent urge to urinate, especially at night.

Individuals with CKD often feel tired or generally weak. This happens because of anemia, a condition characterized by a low red blood cell count due to impaired production of a hormone called erythropoietin, responsible for red blood cell production. Without enough red blood cells to carry oxygen, muscles and the brain can tire quickly.

Swelling or puffiness around the eyes, ankles, feet, or hands can be another sign. This is due to the kidneys' inability to eliminate excess fluid from the body, leading to fluid accumulation in certain areas. Additionally, CKD can result in a poor appetite, a metallic taste in the mouth, or persistent itchy skin caused by the build-up of waste products in the blood.

Early detection of CKD is critical. It not only slows the disease's progression but also helps manage symptoms, thus improving the quality of life for those affected. If you or someone you know is experiencing any of these symptoms, it is essential to consult with a healthcare provider immediately. Remember, CKD often happens alongside other health conditions like diabetes and high blood pressure, so regular health screenings are crucial in early detection and treatment.

Understanding the symptoms of CKD and the importance of early detection is a crucial step toward effectively managing this chronic condition. One can live a healthy and fulfilling life despite a CKD diagnosis through proper dietary modifications, regular check-ups, and following medical advice. This book aims to empower you to protect and care for your kidneys proactively.

1.4. Causes and Risk Factors of Chronic Kidney Disease

Various causes and risk factors can trigger Chronic Kidney Disease (CKD). Understanding these can be crucial in managing the disease and preventing its onset.

Underlying Conditions

The most common causes of CKD are diabetes and high blood pressure. Diabetes mellitus, especially Type 2, often leads to CKD, as high blood sugar levels can damage the kidneys over time. High blood pressure, or hypertension, can also cause CKD as it can strain the glomeruli - the tiny blood vessels in the kidneys where blood is cleaned.

Other conditions that can cause CKD include Glomerulonephritis, a group of diseases that cause inflammation and damage to the kidney's filtering units, and Polycystic kidney disease, a genetic disorder characterized by the growth of numerous cysts in the kidneys. Conditions like Prolonged obstruction of the urinary tract, from conditions like enlarged prostate, kidney stones, and some cancers, Vesicoureteral reflux, a condition that causes urine to back up into your kidneys, and Recurrent kidney infection, also called pyelonephritis, can also lead to CKD.

Risk Factors

Certain risk factors can increase the probability of developing CKD. These include:

- **Age:** CKD is more likely to occur as a person age due to decreased kidney function.
- **Family History:** Those with a family history of kidney disease are more likely to develop CKD.
- **Ethnicity:** Certain ethnic groups, such as African Americans, Native Americans, and Asian Americans, are more prone to CKD, often because of higher rates of diabetes and high blood pressure.
- **Lifestyle Factors:** These include smoking and obesity. Both can increase blood pressure, which is detrimental to kidney health. Lack of physical activity and poor diet, especially a high salt intake, can also contribute to hypertension and CKD.

Medical Conditions

Medical conditions such as cardiovascular disease or other kidney diseases, including hypertension and diabetes, can significantly increase the risk of developing chronic kidney disease (CKD). Individuals with a history of acute kidney injury, such as kidney infections or kidney stones, are also at a higher risk of developing CKD.

Understanding the underlying causes and risk factors of CKD is crucial for taking preventative measures and effectively managing the disease if already diagnosed. It is important to maintain a healthy lifestyle by adopting a balanced diet, engaging in regular physical activity, controlling blood sugar and blood pressure levels, and getting regular check-ups. By proactively addressing these risk factors, individuals can reduce the likelihood of developing CKD or slow its progression, ultimately improving their overall kidney health.

LIKE OUR BOOK? LEAVE A REVIEW!

Enjoyed reading our book? Share your thoughts in writing a review! Scan the QR code to leave your feedback and help others discover the inspiring journey within its pages. Your review matters to us!

2

MAKING SMARTER FOOD CHOICES

P roper nutrition plays a huge role in managing and preventing chronic kidney disease (CKD). Choosing the right foods can help control blood sugar and blood pressure levels, maintain a healthy weight, and reduce complications associated with CKD. Here are some key tips for making smarter food choices to support kidney health:

2.1. Eating Whole and Minimally Processed Foods

Whole and minimally processed foods are the cornerstone of a healthy diet, especially for those managing or preventing chronic kidney disease (CKD). These foods are packed with essential nutrients and lack harmful additives commonly found in heavily processed foods, such as excess salts and sugars. Consuming whole foods can help control blood sugar and blood pressure levels — two crucial factors in kidney health. Moreover, they aid in maintaining a healthy weight, reducing the risk of obesity, another significant risk factor of CKD.

Whole foods come in many forms. **Fruits and vegetables,** for example, are excellent sources of dietary fiber, vitamins, and minerals, with many being low in sodium and high in potassium, essential for kidney health. Examples of kidney-friendly vegetables and fruits include cabbage, red bell pepper, apples, and blueberries.

Whole grains such as brown rice, oatmeal, and whole wheat bread are rich in fiber and B vitamins. They are also known to help maintain healthy cholesterol and blood sugar levels.

Lean proteins, like fish, poultry, and legumes, are essential for building and repairing body tissues. They are also less burdensome on the kidneys compared to their high-fat counterparts.

Finally, **healthy fats,** such as avocados, olives, and nuts, benefit heart health. They can reduce inflammation and lower 'bad' cholesterol levels while raising the 'good' cholesterol levels.

By choosing whole and minimally processed foods, you're ensuring your body — especially your kidneys — receives the nutrients they need without the harmful additives they don't. Furthermore, this dietary change can positively affect your overall health and vitality, making it an excellent lifestyle choice for anyone, not just individuals managing or preventing CKD.

2.2. Detailed List of Kidney-Friendly Whole Foods and Their Benefits

- **Adzuki Beans:** Adzuki beans are low in potassium, making them a great kidney-friendly protein source.
- **Alfalfa Sprouts:** Alfalfa sprouts are low in potassium and high in vitamin K, making them a great addition to a kidney-friendly diet.
- **Almond Butter:** While high in fats, almond butter is lower in potassium and phosphorus than peanut butter, making it a better choice for a kidney diet.

- **Almond Milk:** Almond milk is a delicious and healthier alternative for people with kidney concerns, as it is lower in potassium and phosphorus than dairy.
- **Almonds:** Almonds are a good source of healthy fats, which can help to reduce bad cholesterol (LDL) levels.
- **Apples:** Apples have been known to reduce cholesterol, prevent constipation, protect against heart disease, and reduce cancer risk. They're a good choice for those with kidney disease and are high in fiber and anti-inflammatory properties.
- **Apricot:** Apricots are high in vitamin C and fiber and are good for kidney health due to their low potassium levels.
- **Artichokes:** These vegetables are low in potassium and high in fiber, making them a beneficial addition.
- **Arugula:** This leafy green is low in potassium and high in calcium and antioxidants, making it a good choice for a kidney-friendly diet.
- **Asparagus:** Asparagus is a good source of vitamins A, C, and E, boosting fiber. It's also full of antioxidants.
- **Avocados:** Avocados are rich in healthy fats, fiber, and vitamins, especially B6 and C. They're also a great source maintainhat can help maintain a healthy balance of electrolytes in the body, crucial for kidney health.
- **Barley:** Barley is a fiber-rich grain lower in potassium than other grains.
- **Basil:** This herb is high in antioxidants and low in potassium, making it beneficial for kidney health.
- **Beef:** Lean cuts of beef are lower in potassium and a great protein source.
- **Beets:** Beets are high in antioxidants and beneficial compounds but are lower in potassium than many other vegetables.
- **Bell Peppers:** Bell peppers are low in potassium and high in flavor. They're also an excellent source of vitamin C and vitamin A.

- **Black Beans:** Black beans are an excellent source of plant-based protein and are low in phosphorus, making them a kidney-friendly choice.
- **Blackberries:** Similar to raspberries, blackberries are low in potassium and can provide a sweet-tart flavor.
- **Blackberries:** These berries are low in potassium and high in antioxidants.
- **Blue Crab:** Blue Crab is a good source of lean protein and contains immunity-boosting minerals.
- **Blueberries:** Blueberries are high in antioxidant compounds, which help reduce inflammation and boost immunity. They also contain fiber, vitamin C, vitamin K, and manganese.
- **Broccoli:** Broccoli is high in vitamins C, K, and A, as well as dietary fiber. It also provides anti-inflammatory benefits.
- **Brown Rice:** Brown rice is a whole grain beneficial for kidney health because it is low in sodium and provides dietary fiber, which helps control blood sugar levels, a critical factor in maintaining healthy kidneys.
- **Brussel Sprouts:** Brussel Sprouts are high in fiber, vitamins, minerals, and antioxidants, making them a nutritious addition to your diet.
- **Buckwheat:** Buckwheat is a highly nutritious whole grain with many potential health benefits. It's high in fiber and gluten-free.
- **Bulgur Wheat:** A low-potassium grain that can be used as a rice substitute.
- **Bulgur:** Bulgur is a nutritious whole grain, low in potassium and phosphorus, making it a healthier alternative to other whole grains that are high in these minerals.
- **Butter Lettuce:** This variety of lettuce is low in potassium and adds a delicate buttery taste to salads.
- **Butternut Squash:** Butternut squash is high in vitamins A and C and fiber. It's also a low-potassium alternative to potatoes and other starchy vegetables.

- **Cabbage:** Cabbage is packed with phytochemicals, beneficial compounds that work to break apart free radicals before they can do damage. It's also high in vitamins K and C and a good source of fiber.
- **Canola Oil:** It is a low-potassium, heart-healthy fat option.
- **Cantaloupe:** This melon is lower in potassium than others and can be a refreshing, sweet addition to a kidney-friendly diet.
- **Carrots:** Carrots are rich in beta-carotene, which converts into vitamin A in the body. They also contain antioxidants that promote heart health.
- **Cashew Milk:** Cashew milk is a low-phosphorus, low-potassium milk alternative, making it a good choice for those with kidney issues.
- **Cauliflower:** This versatile vegetable is high in vitamin C and fiber. It's also packed with compounds that help your liver neutralize toxic substances, making it a great choice for kidney health.
- **Celery:** Celery is low in potassium and high in antioxidants, making it a great choice for maintaining good kidney health.
- **Chard:** Swiss chard is lower in potassium than other leafy greens and can be a good addition to a kidney-friendly diet.
- **Cherries:** Cherries have been shown to reduce inflammation when eaten daily. They are also packed with antioxidants and phytochemicals that protect the heart.
- **Chicken Breast:** Chicken breast is a high-quality protein low in potassium, making it a good option for those with kidney issues.
- **Chickpeas:** Chickpeas are high in protein and fiber, making them a filling and nutritious addition to any meal.
- **Cilantro:** Cilantro helps the body eliminate toxins, improving kidney health. It's also a good source of vitamins A, C, and K.
- **Coconut Oil:** While high in saturated fat, it is low in potassium and can be used for cooking at high heat.

- **Cod:** This white fish is lower in potassium than other types and provides a good source of lean protein.
- **Corn:** Corn, particularly sweet corn, is low in potassium and can be a good source of fiber.
- **Cottage Cheese:** This dairy product is lower in potassium than other cheeses and provides a good source of protein.
- **Couscous:** Couscous is low in potassium and can be a great alternative to whole grains high in potassium.
- **Cranberries:** Cranberries are great for preventing urinary tract infections and are packed with vitamin C and fiber.
- **Cranberry Juice:** Pure cranberry juice has antioxidants and can prevent urinary tract infections, helping the kidneys perform better.
- **Cucumber:** Cucumbers are mostly water, making them an excellent hydrating option. They're also low in potassium and high in vitamin K.
- **Cucumbers:** These refreshing vegetables are low in potassium and can be used in salads or as a crunchy snack.
- **Dandelion Greens:** Dandelion greens are full of antioxidants and help to promote good liver and kidney function.
- **Dill:** This is low in potassium and can add flvariousriety of dishes.
- **Dried Cranberries:** Dried cranberries are high in antioxidants and may help to prevent urinary tract infections, which can lead to kidney problems.
- **Egg Whites:** Egg whites are pure protein and provide the highest quality protein with all the essential amino acids. For the kidney diet, egg whites provide protein with less phosphorus than other protein sources such as egg yolk or meats.
- **Eggplant:** Eggplant is a low-potassium vegetable that is beneficial for the kidneys. Grilled or roasted eggplant is a flavorful, low-potassium alternative for side dishes.

- **Endive:** Endive is a low-potassium lettuce alternative that adds a bit of crunch to salads and other dishes.
- **Fennel:** Fennel is a low-potassium vegetable that uniquely flavors dishes.
- **Fig:** Figs are a good dietary fiber source and help keep the kidneys healthy.
- **Fish:** Fish provides high-quality protein and contains anti-inflammatory fats called omega-3s. The healthy fats in fish can help fight diseases such as heart disease and cancer.
- **Flaxseed:** Flaxseed is an excellent source of omega-3 fatty acids and provides anti-inflammatory benefits to the body, including the kidneys.
- **Garlic:** Garlic helps prevent plaque from forming on your teeth, lowers cholesterol, and reduces inflammation. It adds flavor to your dishes and makes them more satisfying without adding harmful sodium.
- **Gooseberries:** Gooseberries are low in potassium and packed with antioxidants, which are good for maintaining kidney health.
- **Grapes:** These juicy fruits are lower in potassium and can be easily incorporated into a kidney-friendly diet.
- **Greek Yogurt:** Greek yogurt is a high-quality source of protein and provides calcium for strong bones.
- **Green Apples:** These fruits are lower in potassium than their red counterparts and can provide a sweet yet tart flavor.
- **Green Beans:** Green beans are a kidney-friendly vegetable due to their lower amount of potassium.
- **Green Peas:** These are lower in potassium than other peas, making them a kidney-friendly option.
- **Green Peppers:** These are lower in potassium than their red and yellow counterparts and add a sweet crunch to meals.
- **Ground Turkey:** Ground turkey, a low-potassium meat option, can be a good source of protein for those with kidney health concerns.

- **Honeydew Melon:** This fruit is low in potassium and can be a refreshing addition to a fruit salad.
- **Jalapenos:** These peppers are low in potassium and can add a spicy kick to your meals.
- **Kale:** Kale is high in vitamins A and C and is a lower-potassium alternative to other leafy greens, beneficial for kidney health.
- **Kelp:** Kelp is a good source of iodine, promoting overall kidney health and preventing thyroid issues.
- **Kiwi:** Kiwi is low in potassium and vitamin C, making it a good fruit choice for a kidney-friendly diet.
- **Leeks:** Leeks are low in potassium and high in flavonoids, which benefit kidney health.
- **Lemon Juice:** Low in potassium, it can be used as a seasoning or in beverages.
- **Lemons:** Lemons are high in vitamin C and help to increase urine volume, helping the kidneys to flush out toxins.
- **Lentils:** Although high in protein and fiber, lentils are lower in potassium than other legumes, making them suitable for a kidney-friendly diet.
- **Lettuce (Iceberg):** Iceberg lettuce is even lower in potassium than other types, making it a good base for salads.
- **Liquid Aminos:** Liquid aminos is a lower-sodium alternative to soy sauce, making it a better choice for those looking to maintain kidney health.
- **Lobster:** This shellfish is low in potassium and can be a good source of lean protein for those on a kidney-friendly diet.
- **Macadamia Nuts:** These nuts, while high in fats, are lower in phosphorus and potassium than other nuts, making them a good choice for a kidney diet.
- **Mackerel:** Mackerel is a high-quality protein source and contains anti-inflammatory omega-3 fatty acids.
- **Maple Syrup:** As a sweetener, maple syrup is low in potassium and a good alternative to honey.
- **Mint:** Mint is a refreshing herb that is low in potassium.

- **Mung Beans:** High in protein and fiber, mung beans are also low in potassium, making them good for kidney health.
- **Mushrooms:** Mushrooms are low in potassium and provide a good source of vitamin D.
- **Mustard Greens:** Mustard greens are rich in vitamins A, K, and C, fiber, and iron. They're also low in potassium.
- **Oatmeal:** Oatmeal is a great source of soluble fiber, which helps to lower cholesterol levels and promote a healthy digestive system.
- **Olive Oil:** Olive oil is a great source of oleic acid, an anti-inflammatory fatty acid. It also contains polyphenols and antioxidant compounds that prevent inflammation and oxidation.
- **Olive Tapenade:** This spread, made from olives, is low in potassium and can add flavor to various dishes.
- **Onion:** Onion is full of flavonoids, particularly quercetin. Flavonoids are natural chemicals that prevent the deposit of fatty materials in blood vessels. Plus, onions are high in vitamin C and a good source of manganese.
- **Oregano:** This herb is not only low in potassium but also packed with antioxidants and can add flavor to a range of dishes.
- **Parsley:** Parsley is rich in antioxidants and may help to reduce kidney inflammation and improve overall kidney function.
- **Pasta:** Whole wheat pasta can be a good source of dietary fiber and is lower in potassium than its whole grain counterpart.
- **Peaches:** Peaches are low in potassium and high in vitamins A and C, making them a kidney-friendly fruit.
- **Pear Barley:** Pear barley is a grain high in fiber but low in potassium and phosphorus, making it beneficial for the kidneys.
- **Pears:** Lower in potassium than other fruits, pears can provide a delicate, sweet flavor.

- **Pine Nuts:** These nuts are lower in phosphorus than others, making them a good choice for a kidney diet.
- **Pineapple Juice:** Pineapple juice is low in potassium and rich in bromelain, aiding kidney health.
- **Pineapple:** A tangy fruit that is rich in fiber, manganese, vitamin C, and bromelain. Pineapples are beneficial for kidney health.
- **Plums:** Plums are lower in potassium than other fruits, making them a good choice for a kidney-friendly diet.
- **Pomegranate Juice:** Pomegranate juice is highly antioxidant and can be a good, low-potassium juice option.
- **Pomegranate:** Pomegranates are packed with antioxidants and can lower inflammation, reduce oxidative stress, and help decrease the risk of kidney disease.
- **Popcorn:** Popcorn is a kidney-friendly snack as long as it's air-popped and lightly seasoned.
- **Portobello Mushrooms:** Portobello mushrooms are an excellent copper, selenium, and niacin source. They're also a great source of protein.
- **Quinoa:** Quinoa is a nutritious seed that has become incredibly popular in the natural health community. It is gluten-free, high in protein, and one of the few plant foods that contain all nine essential amino acids.
- **Radicchio:** Radicchio is a good fiber source, which helps maintain a healthy kidney by preventing constipation and keeping your kidneys healthy.
- **Radish:** Radish is crunchy and hydrating and can help to decrease excess fluids for those with kidney disease. It is also a good source of vitamin C.
- **Raspberries:** These berries are low in potassium and rich in antioxidants, making them a healthy addition to a kidney-friendly diet.
- **Raspberry Leaf Tea:** Raspberry leaf tea can aid in kidney detoxification and is a good source of antioxidants.

- **Red Bell Pepper:** Red bell peppers are low in potassium and high in flavor, but their appeal continues beyond there. They are also an excellent source of vitamins C, A, and B6, fiber, and folic acid. The red hue contains the antioxidant lycopene, known for reducing certain types of cancer.
- **Red Cabbage:** Red cabbage is not only a colorful addition to meals but is also low in potassium.
- **Red Cabbage:** Red cabbage is packed with beneficial compounds and is low in potassium, making it a great choice for a kidney-friendly diet.
- **Red Grapes:** Red grapes and their flavonoids are good for your heart. The skin on red grapes is a particularly rich source of an antioxidant called resveratrol.
- **Red Peppers:** High in vitamin C and low in potassium, red peppers are a good choice for a kidney diet.
- **Red Wine Vinegar:** Red wine vinegar contains acetic acid, which can help aid digestion.
- **Red Wine:** Red wine not only has antioxidants but also can lower the risk of heart disease and inflammation, which can contribute to kidney disease.
- **Rhubarb:** Rhubarb is low in potassium and can be used in various dishes, making it a versatile addition to a kidney-friendly diet.
- **Romaine Lettuce:** Romaine lettuce is a hydrating, low-potassium vegetable high in fiber and vitamin A.
- **Rosemary:** This aromatic herb is high in antioxidants and low in potassium.
- **Salmon:** Salmon is rich in omega-3 fatty acids and reduces inflammation. It's also an excellent source of high-quality protein.
- **Scallions:** Scallions are beneficial for kidney health as they're low in potassium and high in vitamins A and C.
- **Sea Bass:** Sea Bass is a high-quality protein that contains healthy fats called omega-3s. They're good for kidney health because they have anti-inflammatory properties.

- **Seaweed:** Seaweed is a great source of iodine, vitamin K, vitamin B12, and folate and magnesium.
- **Shiitake Mushrooms:** Shiitake mushrooms are an excellent source of vitamins and have powerful antioxidant properties. They also support a healthy immune system.
- **Shrimp:** Shrimp is low in potassium and phosphorus, making it a kidney-friendly seafood option.
- **Spaghetti Squash:** A good low-potassium alternative to traditional pasta.
- **Spinach:** Spinach is packed with vitamins A, C, and K, folate, and iron. It's also low in potassium and beneficial for kidney health.
- **Squash:** Squash is high in vitamins A and C but low in potassium, making it beneficial for those with kidney concerns.
- **Straw Mushrooms:** Like white mushrooms, straw mushrooms are low in potassium and can be used in various dishes.
- **Strawberries:** Strawberries are rich in two types of antioxidants, plus they contain lots of vitamin C, manganese, and fiber. They have anti-inflammatory and anti-cancer properties.
- **Sunflower Seeds:** Sunflower seeds are a good source of protein and monounsaturated and polyunsaturated fats, essential for brain health.
- **Sweet Potatoes:** Sweet potatoes are high in vitamins A and C and are a great source of potassium and fiber. These nutrients boost kidney health by supporting its filtration functions.
- **Swiss Chard:** Swiss chard is packed with kidney-friendly vitamins and minerals, including potassium and magnesium.
- **Tarragon:** This herb is low in potassium and can add a unique, slightly sweet flavor to dishes.

- **Thyme:** This herb is low in potassium and adds a distinctive flavor to a range of dishes.
- **Tofu:** Tofu is a plant-based protein source and provides kidney-friendly protein. It's also low in potassium and high in calcium.
- **Turkey Breast:** Like chicken, turkey breast is low in potassium and a good source of lean protein.
- **Turkey:** Turkey is a high-quality source and low in phosphorus and potassium.
- **Turnips:** Turnips are kidney-friendly as they are low in potassium and phosphorus. They can replace higher-potassium vegetables in many recipes.
- **Turnips:** Turnips are low in potassium and can be baked, boiled, or eaten raw.
- **Vanilla Extract:** A low-potassium flavor enhancer for various dessert recipes.
- **Walnuts:** Walnuts are an excellent source of anti-inflammatory omega-3 fatty acids and are rich in antioxidants. They may help protect against kidney disease by reducing oxidative damage in the body.
- **Water Chestnuts:** These are low in potassium and can add a nice crunch to your salad or stir-fry.
- **Watermelon:** Despite its sweet taste, watermelon is low in potassium and a great option for a refreshing snack or dessert.
- **Wheat Germ:** Wheat germ is packed with important B vitamins, such as folate, thiamin, and vitamin B6, and the minerals zinc and magnesium.
- **White Bread:** As a lower-potassium alternative to whole grain bread, white bread can fit well whole-grain-friendly diet.
- **White Corn:** White corn is low in potassium, making it a better choice for people who need to monitor their potassium intake for kidney health.

- **White Mushrooms:** Compared to other varieties, white mushrooms are lower in potassium, making them a better choice for those with kidney issues.
- **White Rice:** White rice is lower in potassium and phosphorus than brown rice, making it a better choice for a kidney-friendly diet.
- **Zucchini:** Zucchini is low in potassium and high in antioxidants, making it a good option for kidney health.

Incorporating these foods into your diet can support healthy kidney function and prevent or manage kidney disease. Always consult with a healthcare professional before making significant changes to your diet, especially if you have existing health conditions. Furthermore, maintaining a healthy lifestyle.

2.2. Eating Low Glycemic and Anti-Inflammatory Foods

Eating low glycemic and anti-inflammatory foods is crucial for kidney health as it helps control blood sugar levels and reduce inflammation.

Low-glycemic foods are slower to digest and absorb, gradually releasing glucose into the bloodstream. This slow release helps to prevent sudden spikes and drops in blood sugar levels, keeping them stable over time. Maintaining balanced blood sugar levels for kidney health is key, as high levels can strain the kidneys, leading to damage over time. Foods such as whole grains, legumes, and non-starchy vegetables are great examples of low-glycemic foods that can be incorporated into your diet.

On the other hand, anti-inflammatory foods help reduce inflammation, which can negatively impact kidney function if left unchecked. Chronic inflammation may contribute to kidney disease by causing damage to kidney tissue. Foods rich in omega-3 fatty acids, such as fatty fish, walnuts, and flaxseeds, and those high in antioxidants, like berries, spinach, and dark chocolate, have strong anti-inflammatory properties. Incorporating these foods into your diet can help lower inflammation and support kidney health.

Both low glycemic and anti-inflammatory foods benefit kidney health and are cornerstones of a healthy diet, contributing to overall well-being. As always, it is important to consult with a healthcare professional before making any significant dietary changes, especially if you have an underlying health condition. A balanced diet and a healthy lifestyle can significantly improve kidney function and prevent the onset of kidney disease.

Anti-Inflammatory Foods for Kidney Health

- **Almonds:** Almonds are a great source of healthy fats, fiber, and antioxidants, making them a good option for reducing inflammation.
- **Apples:** High in fiber and anti-inflammatory properties, apples help reduce cholesterol, prevent constipation, protect against heart disease, and decrease cancer risk.
- **Apricots:** Apricots are rich in antioxidant vitamins A and C, which help reduce inflammation.
- **Artichokes:** Artichokes are high in antioxidants and contain compounds with anti-inflammatory effects that can help reduce inflammation in the body.
- **Asparagus:** This veggie is an excellent source of anti-inflammatory nutrients and fiber.
- **Avocado:** Avocados are high in monounsaturated fats, which have been shown to have anti-inflammatory effects and may help reduce inflammation in the body.
- **Basil:** Basil contains eugenol, a compound with anti-inflammatory properties that can help decrease inflammation and pain.
- **Beets:** Beets contain betaine, a compound with anti-inflammatory effects that can help reduce inflammation and improve kidney health.

- **Bell Peppers:** Bell peppers are rich in antioxidants and vitamin C, which can help reduce inflammation.
- **Berries:** Berries, including blueberries, strawberries, and raspberries, are packed with antioxidants that can help fight inflammation.
- **Black Beans:** Black beans are a great source of plant-based protein, fiber, and antioxidants that can help lower inflammation.
- **Black Tea:** Black tea has a high concentration of flavonoids and antioxidants that fight inflammation.
- **Blueberries:** Blueberries are packed with antioxidants and vitamin C, which can aid in reducing inflammation. They are also known to help protect the kidneys from damage.
- **Brazil Nuts:** Brazil nuts are an excellent source of selenium, a potent antioxidant that can help reduce inflammation.
- **Broccoli:** Broccoli is a cruciferous vegetable that contains sulforaphane, a compound with anti-inflammatory properties that can help reduce inflammation and protect against various diseases.
- **Broccoli:** Broccoli is high in antioxidants and vitamins that can help fight inflammation.
- **Brown Rice:** Brown rice is a whole grain rich in fiber and antioxidants, making it an excellent choice for reducing inflammation.
- **Brussels Sprouts:** Brussels sprouts are rich in glycosylates, compounds that can help reduce inflammation and protect against certain types of cancer.
- **Buckwheat:** Buckwheat is a whole grain that contains compounds with anti-inflammatory properties.
- **Cabbage:** High in vitamin K, C, and fiber, cabbage is also a good source of vitamin B6 and folic acid. Low in potassium, it's a kidney-friendly cruciferous vegetable.
- **Cantaloupe:** Cantaloupe is high in vitamins A and C, which have anti-inflammatory effects.

- **Carrots:** Carrots are rich in beta-carotene, an antioxidant that has anti-inflammatory effects and may help protect against chronic diseases.
- **Cauliflower:** Cauliflower contains many anti-inflammatory nutrients to help keep inflammation in check.
- **Cauliflower:** Cauliflower is a cruciferous vegetable high in antioxidant and anti-inflammatory compounds, which can help decrease inflammation in the body.
- **Cayenne Pepper:** Cayenne pepper contains capsaicin, a compound known for its anti-inflammatory properties and ability to reduce pain.
- **Celery:** Celery is high in antioxidants and contains compounds with anti-inflammatory effects that can help decrease inflammation in the body.
- **Cherries:** Both sweet and tart cherries are loaded with antioxidants, which can help fight inflammation in the body.
- **Cherries:** Both sweet and tart cherries are packed with antioxidants, which help to reduce inflammation.
- **Chia Seeds:** Chia seeds are a great source of omega-3 fatty acids, antioxidants, and fiber, making them an excellent choice for reducing inflammation.
- **Chickpeas:** Chickpeas are a great source of fiber and plant-based protein, which can help decrease inflammation in the body.
- **Cinnamon:** Cinnamon contains cinnamaldehyde, a compound with powerful antioxidant and anti-inflammatory effects.
- **Citrus Fruits:** Citrus fruits like oranges, lemons, and grapefruits are packed with vitamin C and other anti-inflammatory compounds that can help reduce inflammation.
- **Cloves:** Cloves contain eugenol, a compound with anti-inflammatory effects that can help reduce inflammation and pain.

- **Collard Greens:** Collard greens are rich in antioxidants and have been shown to reduce inflammatory markers in the body.
- **Cranberries:** Cranberries are known for their role in preventing urinary tract infections and are also high in antioxidants and anti-inflammatory compounds, benefiting kidney health.
- **Cucumber:** Cucumbers are high in water and contain compounds with anti-inflammatory properties that may help decrease inflammation and protect against chronic diseases.
- **Dark Chocolate:** Dark chocolate contains flavonoids and antioxidants that can help reduce inflammation and protect against chronic diseases. Choosing dark chocolate with a high cocoa content (70% or higher) is important to reap the most benefits.
- **Dark Chocolate:** Dark chocolate is rich in flavonoids, which have anti-inflammatory effects and can help lower the risk of chronic diseases.
- **Edamame:** Edamame is a good source of plant-based protein and fiber, which can help reduce inflammation.
- **Egg Whites:** Egg whites are pure protein and provide the highest quality of protein with all the essential amino acids, which can help reduce inflammation.
- **Eggplant:** Eggplant is rich in antioxidants and contains compounds with anti-inflammatory effects that can help decrease inflammation in the body.
- **Eggs:** Eggs are rich in choline, a nutrient that can help reduce inflammation.
- **Extra Virgin Olive Oil:** Olive oil is high in oleic acid, an omega-9 fatty acid that can reduce inflammation.
- **Fatty Fish:** Fatty fish like salmon, tuna, and sardines are high in omega-3 fatty acids, which have been shown to have anti-inflammatory effects and may protect against chronic diseases.

- **Fish Oil:** Fish oil is rich in omega-3 fatty acids, known to reduce inflammation. It can be taken as a supplement or consumed through fatty fish.
- **Fish:** Fatty fish like salmon, mackerel, and sardines are high in omega-3 fatty acids, which have been shown to have anti-inflammatory effects and may help protect against chronic diseases.
- **Flaxseeds:** Flaxseeds are high in alpha-linolenic acid (ALA), a type of omega-3 fatty acid that has been shown to reduce inflammation in the body.
- **Flaxseeds:** Flaxseeds are high in omega-3 fatty acids and contain lignans, an antioxidant that can help reduce inflammation.
- **Garbanzo Beans (Chickpeas):** Garbanzo beans are packed with nutrients like protein, fiber, and antioxidants that can help reduce inflammation and protect against chronic diseases.
- **Garlic:** Garlic contains allicin, a compound with anti-inflammatory properties that can help reduce inflammation and protect against chronic diseases.
- **Garlic:** Garlic has been shown to have anti-inflammatory properties, which can help to protect the kidneys.
- **Ginger:** Ginger contains gingerol, a compound with potent anti-inflammatory effects that can help decrease inflammation and oxidative stress.
- **Grapes:** Grapes, particularly red and purple grapes, contain a mix of antioxidants, including flavonoids and resveratrol, which have anti-inflammatory properties.
- **Grapeseed Oil:** Grapeseed oil is high in omega-6 fatty acids and has been linked to reduced inflammation. It's also a healthier cooking oil alternative.
- **Greek Yogurt:** Greek yogurt is rich in probiotics, which can help reduce inflammation in the gut.
- **Green Tea:** Green tea contains a potent antioxidant called epigallocatechin-3-gallate (EGCG), which has anti-

inflammatory effects.

- **Herbs and Spices:** Herbs and spices like rosemary, thyme, oregano, cinnamon, and cloves contain high levels of antioxidants and anti-inflammatory compounds that can help reduce inflammation.
- **Kale:** Kale, another nutrient-dense leafy green, is high in antioxidants and anti-inflammatory compounds that help protect against chronic diseases and improve kidney health.
- **Kefir:** Kefir is a fermented dairy product that can help reduce inflammation.
- **Kombucha:** Kombucha is a fermented drink that's rich in probiotics and can help reduce inflammation in the gut.
- **Leeks:** Leeks are a good source of kaempferol, a natural flavonol known to have anti-inflammatory properties.
- **Lentils:** Lentils are high in protein, fiber, and antioxidants like polyphenols that have anti-inflammatory effects.
- **Mackerel:** Mackerel is a fatty fish high in omega-3 fatty acids, known for their anti-inflammatory effects.
- **Mangoes:** Mangoes contain a complex mix of polyphenols with anti-inflammatory properties.
- **Miso:** Miso is a fermented soy product high in probiotics and can help decrease inflammation.
- **Mushrooms:** Mushrooms contain compounds like beta-glucans and ergothioneine, which have been shown to have anti-inflammatory effects on the body. They also contain antioxidants that can help reduce inflammation.
- **Nuts and Seeds:** Nuts and seeds like almonds, walnuts, chia seeds, and flaxseeds are high in omega-3 fatty acids, antioxidants, and other compounds that can help reduce inflammation in the body.
- **Oats:** Oats are high in fiber and contain compounds that have been shown to reduce inflammation in the body.
- **Olive Oil:** Olive oil is high in monounsaturated fats and contains compounds with anti-inflammatory effects that can help reduce inflammation in the body.

- **Onions:** Onions are high in vitamin C, manganese, and prebiotic fiber that help keep your gut healthy.
- **Oranges:** Oranges are packed with vitamin C, a potent antioxidant that helps reduce inflammation.
- **Oregano:** Oregano contains carvacrol and thymol, compounds with anti-inflammatory effects that can help decrease inflammation in the body.
- **Papaya:** Papaya is rich in antioxidants like vitamin C and beta-carotene, making it a great choice for reducing inflammation.
- **Parsley:** Parsley is rich in antioxidants that can help fight inflammation.
- **Peaches:** Peaches have antioxidant and anti-inflammatory properties, thanks to their vitamins A and C content.
- **Pineapple:** Pineapple contains bromelain, an enzyme with anti-inflammatory properties that can help reduce pain and swelling in conditions like arthritis.
- **Pistachios:** Pistachios are rich in healthy fats and contain inflammation-fighting antioxidants.
- **Pomegranate:** Pomegranates contain antioxidants and anti-inflammatory properties, which may help improve kidney health.
- **Probiotic-rich Foods:** Probiotics are beneficial bacteria that can help improve gut health and reduce inflammation. Foods like yogurt, kefir, sauerkraut, and kimchi are good sources of probiotics.
- **Pumpkin Seeds:** Pumpkin seeds are a good source of magnesium, zinc, and other nutrients that can help decrease inflammation.
- **Quinoa:** Quinoa is a whole grain high in antioxidants and fiber, making it an excellent anti-inflammatory food.
- **Radishes:** They are crunchy, hydrating, and packed with anti-inflammatory properties. They can be eaten raw, cooked, or pickled.

- **Raspberries:** Raspberries are delicious and packed with antioxidants and anti-inflammatory compounds, which can help maintain healthy kidneys.
- **Red Bell Peppers:** Red bell peppers are low in potassium and high in flavor. They're also packed with vitamins C, A, B6, folic acid, and fiber, which can help reduce inflammation.
- **Red cabbage:** Red cabbage contains antioxidants, including flavonoids and sulfur compounds, which offer anti-inflammatory benefits.
- **Red Grapes:** Red grapes, rich in resveratrol, a type of flavonoid, have potent anti-inflammatory effects that can support healthy kidneys.
- **Red Wine:** Red wine contains resveratrol, a compound with anti-inflammatory properties that can help decrease inflammation and protect against chronic diseases.
- **Rosemary:** Rosemary contains rosmarinic acid, a compound with anti-inflammatory properties that can help reduce inflammation.
- **Salmon:** Salmon is a fatty fish high in omega-3 fatty acids, making it an excellent choice for reducing inflammation.
- **Sardines:** Sardines are another type of fatty fish high in omega-3 fatty acids and can help reduce inflammation.
- **Sauerkraut:** Sauerkraut is a fermented cabbage dish rich in probiotics that can help reduce gut inflammation.
- **Shiitake Mushrooms:** Shiitake mushrooms contain compounds like eritadenine, which has been shown to have anti-inflammatory properties and may improve immune function.
- **Soy Products:** Soy products like tofu, tempeh, and soy milk are high in isoflavones, antioxidants that have been shown to decrease inflammation in the body.
- **Spinach:** Spinach is high in antioxidants and vitamin A that can help reduce inflammation and protect kidney health.

- **Spirulina:** Spirulina is a blue-green algae with antioxidants that can help reduce inflammation.
- **Strawberries:** Strawberries are high in antioxidants and vitamin C, which can help reduce inflammation and improve kidney health.
- **Sunflower Seeds:** Sunflower seeds are a good source of vitamin E and other antioxidants to help decrease inflammation.
- **Sweet Potatoes:** Sweet potatoes are rich in beta-carotene, an antioxidant that can help decrease inflammation and protect against chronic diseases.
- **Tempeh:** Tempeh is a fermented soy product high in protein and probiotics, which can help decrease inflammation.
- **Tofu:** Tofu is a soy product, and soy has been shown to reduce inflammation.
- **Tomatoes:** Tomatoes are rich in lycopene, an antioxidant that has been shown to have anti-inflammatory properties and may help protect against chronic diseases.
- **Turmeric:** Turmeric contains curcumin, a compound with strong anti-inflammatory effects that has been shown to improve kidney health and protect against chronic diseases.
- **Walnuts:** Walnuts are a good source of plant-based omega-3 fatty acids and polyphenols, which have anti-inflammatory effects.
- **Water:** Staying hydrated is important for the kidneys and overall health. Water helps flush out toxins and waste products from the body, reducing inflammation and improving kidney function.
- **Watermelon:** Watermelon is rich in antioxidants and provides hydration, which can reduce inflammation.
- **Whole Grains:** Whole grains like quinoa, brown rice, and oats are high in fiber and other compounds that can help decrease inflammation and improve gut health.
- **Yogurt:** Yogurt is high in probiotics, which can help decrease inflammation in the gut and improve overall health.

- **Zucchini:** Zucchini is high in antioxidants and anti-inflammatory phytonutrients.

As you can see, plenty of delicious and nutritious foods can help fight inflammation in the body. Incorporating these anti-inflammatory foods into your diet can support your overall health and potentially reduce the risk of chronic diseases. Maintaining a balanced and varied diet, including various fruits, vegetables, healthy fats, and lean proteins, is important.

Additionally, avoiding processed and high-sugar foods can also help reduce inflammation in the body. Food is our fuel, so choose wisely to support a healthy, inflammation-free lifestyle. So, next time you plan your meals, consider adding some anti-inflammatory foods for a tasty and beneficial boost!

2.3. Avoiding High Glycemic and Inflammatory Foods

- **Alcohol:** Alcohol can cause an inflammatory response in the body, especially when consumed excessively.
- **Artificial Juices:** High in sugar and often containing artificial flavors, these juices can cause inflammation.
- **Artificial Sweeteners and Additives:** Certain food additives and artificial sweeteners can trigger an inflammatory response in some people.
- **Bagels:** Bagels made from refined flour can cause a spike in blood sugar levels, leading to inflammation.
- **Bagged Snack Foods:** Foods like potato chips and cheesy puff snacks are high in trans fats and sodium, leading to inflammation.
- **Baked Goods:** Pastries, cakes, and cookies are often made with refined flour and sugar, which can contribute to inflammation. Limit your intake of these treats and opt for healthier homemade versions using whole-grain flour and natural sweeteners.

- **BBQ Sauce:** BBQ sauce is often high in sugar and sodium, leading to inflammation.
- **Biscuits and Pastries:** These are often made with refined flour, unhealthy fats, and added sugars, contributing to inflammation.
- **Bottled Salad Dressings:** Many bottled salad dressings contain added sugars and unhealthy fats, leading to inflammation.
- **Bottled Smoothies:** While they may seem healthy, many bottled smoothies contain added sugars and unhealthy additives, contributing to inflammation.
- **Bottled:** Like fruit juice, bottled tea often contains added sugars that can increase inflammation.
- **Breaded Chicken:** Fried and breaded chicken is high in unhealthy fats and can trigger inflammation.
- **Brown Sugar:** Like white sugar, consuming too much brown sugar can lead to inflammation.
- **Cakes with Frosting:** The cake and the frosting are high in sugar unhealthy fats and can trigger inflammation.
- **Cakes:** High in sugar and fat, most cakes can lead to inflammation.
- **Candied Nuts:** This snack's added sugar and unhealthy fats can trigger inflammation.
- **Candies:** Candies are usually loaded with sugar and artificial ingredients that can contribute to inflammation.
- **Candy and Chocolates:** High in sugar and fat, these treats can cause inflammation.
- **Candy Bars** are high in sugar and unhealthy fats that can trigger an inflammatory response.
- **Canned Beans with added salt:** Canned vegetables, beans with added sauces can be high in sodium and preservatives, leading to inflammation.
- **Canned Chili:** Usually high in sodium and often made with unhealthy fats, canned chili can cause inflammation.

- **Canned Frostings** are high in sugar and unhealthy fats, contributing to inflammation.
- **Canned Fruit in Heavy Syrup:** The high sugar content from the syrup can contribute to inflammation.
- **Canned Fruit in Syrup:** Packed with added sugars, canned fruit in syrup can cause a spike in blood sugar levels and contribute to inflammation.
- **Canned Soup:** Canned soups are typically high in sodium and preservatives, which can lead to inflammation.
- **Canned Vegetables with Added Salt:** Canned vegetables are often high in sodium, which can contribute to inflammation.
- **Canned Vegetables with Added Sauce:** Many canned vegetables have added sa are high in sodium and preservatives, leading to inflammation.
- **Canned Vegetables:** Often high in sodium and preservatives, canned vegetables can contribute to inflammation.
- **Caramel Popcorn:** The sugar and butter content in caramel popcorn can lead to inflammation.
- **Cereal Bars:** While marketed as a healthy snack, many cereal bars are high in added sugars and unhealthy fats, leading to inflammation.
- **Cheese:** Certain types of cheese, especially processed cheese, can trigger inflammation.
- **Cheeseburgers:** High in unhealthy fats and often served with refined bread, this can lead to inflammation.
- **Chips and Snack Mixes:** These snacks often contain trans fats and high sodium levels, leading to inflammation.
- **Chips:** Fried and often made with inflammatory vegetable oils, chips can trigger inflammation.
- **Commercial Baked Goods:** Packaged cookies, cakes, and other baked goods are usually high in added sugars and unhealthy fats, leading to inflammation.
- **Commercial BBQ Sauce:** Store-bought BBQ sauces are often high in sugar and preservatives, which can trigger inflammation.

- **Commercial Cookies:** Packaged cookies are often high in sugar and unhealthy fats, which can trigger inflammation.
- **Commercial Smoothies:** Often high in added sugars, commercial smoothies can cause inflammation.
- **Condiments with Added Sugar:** Many condiments, such as ketchup and BBQ sauce, contain added sugars that can contribute to inflammation.
- **Cookies:** Full of sugar and unhealthy fats, cookies can contribute to inflammation.
- **Corn Syrup:** This sweetener is high in fructose, leading to inflammation.
- **Cotton Candy:** Pure sugar spun into a fluffy treat; cotton candy can lead to inflammation.
- **Cough Syrups:** Many cough syrups are high in added sugars, which can lead to inflammation.
- **Crackers:** Often made with refined flour and high in sodium, crackers can trigger inflammation.
- **Cream Cheese:** Cream cheese is high in saturated fats and can contribute to inflammation.
- **Cream-based Salad Dressings:** These are often high in unhealthy fats and can trigger inflammation.
- **Crispy Fried Onion Rings:** Deep-fried and high in unhealthy fats, onion rings can contribute to inflammation.
- **Cupcakes:** Cupcakes are often high in sugar unhealthy fats, and made from refined flour.
- **Deep Fried Foods:** Foods like fried chicken and fried potatoes are high in unhealthy fats and can cause inflammation.
- **Deli Meats:** Processed deli meats often contain preservatives high in sodium, leading to inflammation.
- **Donuts:** Donuts are typically high in sugar and trans fats, contributing to inflammation.
- **Dried Fruit:** Although natural sources of sugar, dried fruits are often packed with added sugars that can trigger inflammation in the body.

- **Energy Drinks:** These beverages are often loaded with sugar and unhealthy additives that can cause inflammation.
- **Fast Food Burgers:** High in unhealthy fats sodium, and often served with a refined flour bun, fast food burgers can lead to inflammation.
- **Fast Food:** Highly processed and often loaded with unhealthy additives, fast food can contribute to inflammation in the body. Limit your intake of these foods and choose healthier options when dining out.
- **Flavored Coffee Drinks:** Coffee drinks with high sugar levels and artificial flavorings can cause inflammation.
- **Flavored Instant Oatmeal:** Like instant oatmeal, flavored varieties are often high in added sugars and unhealthy additives that can cause inflammation.
- **Flavored Potato Chips:** Like regular chips, flavored potato chips are often fried and contain inflammatory vegetable oils.
- **Flavored Waters:** Like energy drinks, flavored waters are often high in added sugars and unhealthy additives that can cause inflammation.
- **Flavored Yogurt:** Many flavored yogurts are high in sugar, which can increase inflammation.
- **French Fries:** Typically deep-fried, French fries are high in unhealthy fats and can cause inflammation.
- **Fried Chicken:** High in unhealthy fats and often coated in refined flour, fried chicken can trigger inflammation.
- **Fried Foods:** Foods that are fried, especially in unhealthy oils, can cause inflammation.
- **Frozen Breakfast Burritos:** Like frozen breakfast sandwiches, these burritos are often high in processed meats, sodium, and preservatives that can trigger inflammation.
- **Frozen Breakfast Sandwiches:** Like processed meats, frozen breakfast sandwiches are often high in sodium and preservatives that can cause inflammation.

- **Frozen Chicken Nuggets:** Often made with refined flour and high in unhealthy fats, frozen chicken nuggets can lead to inflammation.
- **Frozen Dinners:** Many frozen meals are high in sodium and contain preservatives, which can increase inflammation.
- **Frozen Fish Sticks:** Usually high in sodium and preservatives, frozen fish sticks can trigger inflammation.
- **Frozen Meals:** Most frozen meals contain high amounts of sodium and preservatives, which can cause inflammation.
- **Frozen Pizza:** Similar to store-bought pizza, frozen pizza is often high in sodium and unhealthy fats that can contribute to inflammation.
- **Frozen TV Dinners:** These convenience meals are often high in sodium, unhealthy fats, and preservatives, triggering inflammation.
- **Frozen Waffles with Syrup:** The combination of refined flour in waffles and the high sugar content in syrup can cause inflammation.
- **Fruit Jams:** Many fruit jams are high in added sugars, which can lead to inflammation.
- **Fruit Juice:** While natural fruit juice may seem healthy, it often contains added sugars that can contribute to inflammation.
- **Fruit Punch:** High in sugar and often containing artificial flavors, fruit punch can cause inflammation.
- **Fruit Snacks:** Often marketed as a healthy snack, fruit snacks are typically high in added sugars that can cause inflammation.
- **Fruit Yogurts:** While yogurt can be healthy, high-sugar versions can lead to inflammation.
- **Fruit-flavored Yogurt:** Like sugary yogurt, fruit-flavored yogurts are often high in added sugars and can trigger inflammation.
- **Gelato:** This sweet treat is high in sugar, which can lead to inflammation.

- **Glazed Donuts:** High in sugar and unhealthy fats, these treats can trigger inflammation.
- **High-Fructose Corn Syrup:** This common sweetener is often found in packaged foods and beverages, contributing to inflammation.
- **Highly Processed Foods:** Foods that are highly processed, like ready-made meals or snack foods, often contain unhealthy fats and added sugars, both of which can lead to inflammation.
- **High-Sugar Cereals:** Many cereals marketed towards children are high in added sugars, which can trigger inflammation.
- **Honey:** Despite its health benefits, too much honey can lead to inflammation due to its high sugar content.
- **Hot Dogs:** These processed meats are high in unhealthy fats, sodium, and preservatives, which can increase inflammation.
- **Hydrogenated Oils:** These oils contain trans fats, which can lead to inflammation.
- **Ice Cream:** This dessert, especially the commercial variants, is high in sugar and unhealthy fats, which can cause inflammation.
- **Instant Breakfast Drinks:** Like energy drinks, instant breakfast drinks are often high in added sugars and unhealthy additives that can trigger inflammation.
- **Instant Macaroni and Cheese:** This convenience food is high in sodium and contains refined flour, contributing to inflammation.
- **Instant Mashed Potatoes:** Made from refined potatoes and often loaded with unhealthy additives, instant mashed potatoes can contribute to inflammation.
- **Instant Noodles:** High in sodium and often made with refined flour, instant noodles can contribute to inflammation.
- **Instant Oatmeal:** While it may seem like a healthy breakfast option, instant oatmeal is often high in added sugars and

unhealthy additives that can cause inflammation.

- **Instant Pudding:** The added sugars and unhealthy fats in instant pudding can contribute to inflammation.
- **Instant Ramen Noodles:** High in sodium and made with refined flour, instant ramen noodles can trigger inflammation in the body.
- **Instant Ramen:** Instant ramen is usually high in sodium and contains unhealthy additives, which can increase inflammation.
- **Jams and Jellies:** These spreads are typically high in added sugars, contributing to inflammation.
- **Jelly and Jam:** High in added sugars, these can contribute to inflammation.
- **Jelly Candies:** Jelly candies are pure sugar and can cause inflammation.
- **Ketchup:** Ketchup can contain high amounts of sugar and sodium, contributing to inflammation.
- **Maple Syrup:** Pure maple syrup is high in sugar and can lead to inflammation.
- **Margarine:** Often made with unhealthy vegetable oils, margarine can cause inflammation in the body.
- **Marshmallows:** These are high in sugar, leading to inflammation.
- **Mayonnaise:** Mayonnaise can be high in unhealthy fats, leading to inflammation.
- **Microwave Popcorn:** Often loaded with unhealthy additives, microwave popcorn can contribute to inflammation.
- **Microwaveable Breakfast Sandwiches:** These convenience foods are often high in sodium, unhealthy fats, and refined flour, contributing to inflammation.
- **Milk Chocolate:** While dark chocolate has anti-inflammatory properties, milk chocolate is usually high in added sugars and unhealthy fats, leading to inflammation.
- **Muffins:** Muffins, especially those commercially made, are often high in sugar and unhealthy fats.

- **Non-dairy Coffee Creamers:** These often contain trans fats and high-fructose corn syrup, which can lead to inflammation.
- **Packaged Cheese:** Like processed cheese, packaged cheese slices are often high in sodium and preservatives that can cause inflammation.
- **Packaged Desserts:** These are often high in sugars and unhealthy fats and contain preservatives, contributing to inflammation.
- **Packaged Macaroni and Cheese:** Often high in sodium and unhealthy fats, packaged macaroni and cheese can contribute to inflammation.
- **Packaged Muffins:** Often high in added sugars and unhealthy fats, packaged muffins can contribute to inflammation.
- **Pancakes with Syrup:** The combination of refined flour in pancakes and the high sugar content in syrup can cause inflammation.
- **Pastries, Cakes, and Cookies:** These sweet treats are typically high in sugar, unhealthy fats, and refined flour, making them high on the glycemic index and pro-inflammatory.
- **Peanut Butter:** Some peanut butter brands contain added sugar and unhealthy oils, contributing to inflammation.
- **Pepperoni Pizza:** This popular food item is high in unhealthy fats and sodium, which can trigger inflammation.
- **Pies:** Pies are typically high in sugar and unhealthy fats and are made from refined flour.
- **Pizza:** Commercially available pizzas are often made with refined flour and are high in sodium, unhealthy fats, and preservatives, leading to inflammation.
- **Pop Tarts:** High in sugar and refined flour, pop tarts can cause a spike in blood sugar levels and contribute to inflammation.

- **Popcorn:** While popcorn can be a healthy snack, versions that are high in salt, butter, or sugar can lead to inflammation.
- **Popsicles:** Popsicles are typically high in sugar, which can cause inflammation.
- **Potato Chips:** High in trans fats and often containing artificial flavors, potato chips can cause inflammation.
- **Potatoes:** While nutritious in moderation, potatoes have a high glycemic index and can cause inflammation when consumed in excess.
- **Powdered Sugar:** This type of sugar can spike blood sugar levels and cause inflammation.
- **Pre-made Pies and Pastries:** These are typically high in sugar unhealthy fats, and made from refined flour, all contributing to inflammation.
- **Pretzels:** Made from refined grains, pretzels can cause a spike in blood sugar levels and contribute to inflammation.
- **Processed Breakfast Cereals:** Many breakfast cereals are high in added sugars and refined grains, contributing to inflammation.
- **Processed Cheese:** High in sodium and often containing preservatives, processed cheese can trigger inflammation.
- **Processed Cheese:** High in sodium and preservatives, processed cheese can contribute to inflammation in the body.
- **Processed Frozen Meals:** Similar to frozen pizzas and breakfast burritos, frozen meals are often high in sodium and unhealthy fats that can contribute to inflammation. Opt for homemade or fresh meals instead.
- **Processed Meats:** Deli meats, bacon, and other processed meats are often high in sodium and preservatives that can trigger inflammation. Opt for fresh cuts of meat or plant-based protein sources as a healthier option.
- **Processed Snack Bars:** Many snack bars are marketed as healthy options but are often high in added sugars and

unhealthy additives that can contribute to inflammation.

- **Processed Vegetable Oils:** Vegetable oils like canola and soybean oil are often highly processed and contain inflammatory compounds.
- **Puffed Rice:** Having a high glycemic index, puffed rice can contribute to inflammation.
- **Ramen:** While delicious, ramen is often high in refined carbohydrates, sodium, and unhealthy fats.
- **Red and Processed Meats:** These types of meats are high in saturated fat, which can lead to inflammation.
- **Refined Cereals:** Highly processed cereals typically contain added sugars and lack fiber, which can contribute to inflammation.
- **Regular Soda:** High in sugar of any nutritional benefits, regular soda can cause a spike in blood sugar levels, leading to inflammation.
- **Rice Cakes:** White rice cakes have a high glycemic index and can trigger inflammation.
- **Rice Puddings:** These are high in sugar and can cause inflammation.
- **Sauces and Marinades with Added Sugars:** Many packaged sauces and marinades contain added sugars, which can contribute to inflammation in the body. Opt for homemade versions using natural sweeteners or options with no added sugars.
- **Sausages:** Sausages often contain high levels of salt and preservatives, contributing to inflammation.
- **Sherbet:** Sherbet is high in sugar, leading to inflammation.
- **Soda:** Carbonated beverages are typically loaded with sugars, making them a cause of inflammation.
- **Sodas:** Loaded with sugar and unhealthy additives, sodas can trigger inflammation in the body.
- **Soft Drinks:** These drinks are typically high in sugar, leading to inflammation.

- **Soy Sauce:** Soy sauce is high in sodium, which can lead to inflammation.
- **Spaghetti:** Spaghetti, especially those made from refined wheat, can lead to inflammation.
- **Store-bought Cakes and Muffins:** These are typically high in sugar, made with refined flour, and contain unhealthy fats, contributing to inflammation.
- **Store-bought Granola Bars:** Many commercial granola bars are high in sugar and unhealthy additives, which can cause inflammation.
- **Store-bought Pasta Sauce:** Like condiments, many store-bought pasta sauces contain added sugars that can trigger inflammation.
- **Store-bought Salad Dressing:** Many store-bought salad dressings are high in added sugars and unhealthy fats, contributing to inflammation.
- **Store-bought Smoothies:** Often marketed as a healthy option, many store-bought smoothies are high in added sugars and unhealthy additives, leading to inflammation.
- **Sugar-sweetened Beverages:** Drinks high in sugar, such as sodas and fruit juices, can cause inflammation and are also high on the glycemic index.
- **Sugary Alcoholic Beverages:** Cocktails and other alcoholic beverages are often filled with added sugars that can trigger inflammation. Opt for drinks with no added sugars or limit your intake to reduce inflammation.
- **Sugary Breakfast Cereals:** These cereals are high in sugar and low in fiber, which can trigger inflammation.
- **Sugary Cereals:** Many cereals marketed towards children are high in added sugars, which can trigger inflammation in the body. Instead, choose whole grain options with no added sugars for a healthier breakfast.
- **Sugary Coffee Drinks:** Many coffee drinks, such as flavored lattes and frappuccinos, are loaded with added sugars that can cause inflammation in the body. Stick to plain coffee or

tea with minimal or no added sugar to avoid triggering inflammation.

- **Sugary Drinks:** Sodas, sweetened teas, and other sugary beverages are loaded with added sugars that can cause inflammation in the body. Instead, opt for water or unsweetened tea as a healthier alternative.
- **Sugary Energy Drinks:** While marketed as energy source energy, many energy drinks are high in added sugars and unhealthy additives that can cause inflammation.
- **Sugary Granola Bars:** Despite their healthy image, many granola bars are high in sugar and can lead to inflammation.
- **Sugary Iced Tea:** While iced tea can be a healthy drink, high-sugar versions can lead to inflammation.
- **Sugary Snack Bars:** While marketed as a healthy snack, many granola and energy bars are high in added sugars that can trigger inflammation. Choose options with minimal or no added sugars for a healthier option.
- **Sugary Yogurt:** Flavored yogurt is often filled with added sugars that can cause inflammation. Opt for plain Greek yogurt and add fresh fruit for a healthier option.
- **Sweetened Almond Milk:** It often contains added sugars, which can cause inflammation.
- **Sweetened Coffee Drinks:** Like energy drinks, sweetened coffee drinks are often high in added sugars and unhealthy additives that can cause inflammation.
- **Sweetened Condensed Milk:** Its high sugar content can cause inflammation.
- **Sweetened Dried Fruits:** The additional sugar in sweetened dried fruits can lead to inflammation.
- **Sweetened Flavored Milk:** The added sugars in these drinks can lead to inflammation.
- **Sweetened Iced Tea:** Iced tea that contains added sugar can lead to inflammation.
- **Sweetened Yogurt:** While yogurt can be healthy, versions that are high in sugar can lead to inflammation.

- **Table Salt:** Consumed in excess, table salt can contribute to inflammation in the body.
- **Tortillas:** Made from refined wheat, tortillas can lead to inflammation.
- **Vegetable Chips:** While they seem a healthier option, vegetable chips are often fried and contain inflammatory vegetable oils.
- **White Bagels:** White bagels are made from refined flour, which can spike blood sugar levels and cause inflammation.
- **White Bread:** White bread is made from refined wheat, which is high in the glycemic index and can lead to inflammation.
- **White Pasta and Rice:** These high-glycemic foods can cause a spike in blood sugar levels and contribute to inflammation.
- **White Pasta:** Made from refined flour, white pasta can cause a rise in blood sugar levels and contribute to inflammation.
- **White Rice:** Like white bread, white rice is made from refined grains and can cause a spike in blood sugar levels, contributing to inflammation.
- **White Sugar:** Highly processed and devoid of any nutritional value, white sugar can increase inflammation in the body.

As the list shows, many processed foods can contribute to inflammation in the body. It is important to read labels and make conscious decisions about what we put into our bodies. Choosing whole, unprocessed foods can help reduce the risk of inflammation and promote overall health. In addition to avoiding inflammatory foods, incorporating anti-inflammatory foods into our diet, such as fruits and vegetables, can also help combat inflammation. By being mindful of our food choices, we can work towards reducing inflammation and improving our overall well-being. Avoiding these foods can lower your glycemic index and reduce inflammation, thereby supporting your overall health and well-being.

3

MANAGING DIABETES AND KIDNEY HEALTH

D iabetes and kidney health are closely related, as diabetes is one of the leading causes of chronic kidney disease. Approximately 1 in 3 people with diabetes will develop some form of kidney disease in their lifetime. This is why it is important for individuals with diabetes to actively manage their blood sugar levels and monitor their kidney function.

3.1. The Glycemic Index Diet Explained

The Glycemic Index (GI) ranks carbohydrate-containing foods based on how they affect blood sugar levels. Foods are scored on a scale of 0 to 100, with pure glucose being 100. Foods with a high GI (70 or above) are rapidly digested and absorbed, causing a quick and significant spike in blood sugar levels. On the other hand, foods with a low GI (55 or below) are digested and absorbed at a slower pace, resulting in a gradual rise in blood sugar levels.

Why is this important for kidney health? Among their other functions, our kidneys help regulate blood glucose levels by filtering and reabsorbing glucose. When one consistently consumes high-GI foods, it can lead to perpetual high blood sugar levels, also known as hyperglycemia. Over time, hyperglycemia can damage the tiny blood vessels in the kidneys, impairing their ability to effectively filter waste from the blood. This condition is known as diabetic nephropathy, a serious consequence of unmanaged diabetes.

Opting for a diet rich in low-GI foods can help manage blood sugar levels more effectively, reducing the risk of hyperglycemia and its associated complications. Foods such as whole grains, legumes, fruits, and non-starchy vegetables are all excellent choices for a low-GI diet. By understanding and implementing the principles of a low-GI diet, individuals can take an active role in managing their diabetes and supporting their kidney health.

Remember, a low-GI diet is not about restricting certain foods but understanding how different foods can impact your blood sugar levels and making informed choices. Always consult a healthcare provider before making any significant changes to your diet. In a world where diet trends come and go, the GI diet remains a scientifically supported approach to managing blood sugar levels and promoting kidney health.

Understanding the Value of the Glycemic Index in Managing Diabetes

The Glycemic Index (GI) diet is a powerful tool in managing diabetes, primarily because it encourages an understanding of how different foods impact blood sugar levels. The diet's core premise is about what you eat and how the body metabolizes these foods.

Let's delve deeper into the mechanics of it all. Foods with a high GI rapidly raise blood glucose levels, prompting the body to release insulin. However, in individuals with diabetes, this mechanism is either faulty, causing hyperglycemia (type 1 diabetes), or the body's cells are resistant to insulin, leading to a surplus of glucose in the blood (type 2 diabetes). Consistently high blood sugar levels can cause severe complications, including diabetic nephropathy, as mentioned earlier.

On the other hand, consuming foods with a lower GI results in slower absorption and a more gradual increase in blood glucose levels. This reduces the need for insulin secretion, making it easier to manage blood glucose levels, particularly for individuals with type 2 diabetes.

Incorporating a low-GI diet into your life can be as simple as swapping white bread for whole-grain bread or choosing steel-cut oats over instant oats for breakfast. These choices can make a significant difference in blood sugar management.

However, it's essential to remember that the GI of food is not the only factor to consider when making dietary choices. Nutritional balance, portion sizes, and personal preferences also play a considerable role in creating a sustainable and effective meal plan for managing diabetes. Moreover, not all low-GI foods are necessarily healthy (chocolate, for instance, has a low GI), and not all high-GI foods should be avoided (watermelon, despite its high GI, is highly nutritious).

The real value of the GI diet comes from using it as a guide to make healthier food choices, leading to stable blood sugar levels and, thus, better management of diabetes. Always consult with a healthcare provider or a dietician before making significant changes to your diet. By understanding and implementing these principles, individuals can gain control over their diabetes, improve their overall health, and enhance their quality of life.

3.2. Low-Glycemic Diet and Your Health

Adopting a low-GI diet involves more than selecting the right foods; it's about integrating mindful habits into your daily routine. Here are some practical steps to get you started:

1. **Be Informed:** Knowledge is the first step. Familiarize yourself with the GI values of common foods. Reference charts are available online and in various health books.
2. **Choose Whole Foods:** Whole, unprocessed foods are generally lower in GI. Opt for whole grains, fruits, vegetables, and lean proteins.
3. **Swap High-GI Foods:** Simple switches can make a big difference. Replace white rice with brown rice or quinoa, and swap potato chips with nuts or seeds for a snack.
4. **Combine Foods:** Consuming high-GI foods with protein or healthy fats can help slow the absorption of sugar into your bloodstream and prevent spikes in insulin.
5. **Practice Portion Control:** Large meals can cause blood sugar spikes, even if the food is low-GI. Pay attention to serving sizes to avoid overeating.
6. **Stay Hydrated:** Regular water intake is essential for overall health and can help control blood sugar and appetite.
7. **Exercise Regularly:** Physical activity helps your body use insulin more effectively and can lower blood sugar levels.

Remember, transitioning to a low-GI diet isn't about adhering to strict dietary limitations or depriving yourself of the foods you love. It's about creating a balanced, sustainable lifestyle that enhances health and well-being. Always consult a healthcare provider before making any significant changes to your diet. By incorporating these tips, you'll be well on your way to reaping the benefits of a low-GI diet.

The Impact of a Low-GI Diet on Kidney Health

The kidneys play a critical role in maintaining overall health by filtering waste products from the blood. However, conditions like diabetes can strain these vital organs, potentially leading to kidney disease or kidney failure. A low-GI diet can substantially benefit kidney health, particularly for individuals with diabetes.

Firstly, a low-GI diet assists in managing blood sugar levels, reducing the kidney burden. When blood sugar levels are consistently high due to diabetes, the kidneys have to work harder to filter the blood, which can lead to kidney damage over time. By promoting stable blood glucose levels, a low-GI diet helps to alleviate this stress on the kidneys.

In addition, a low-GI diet's focus on whole, unprocessed foods can support kidney health in other ways. These foods are often rich in nutrients like potassium, magnesium, and fiber, contributing to healthy kidney function. Furthermore, many low-GI foods are low in sodium, a mineral that, when consumed in excess, can put pressure on the kidneys and contribute to hypertension, a significant risk factor for kidney disease.

Also, by encouraging portion control, a low-GI diet can help prevent obesity, another risk factor for kidney disease. Maintaining a healthy weight reduces the strain on the kidneys and helps them perform their vital functions more effectively.

In summary, a low-GI diet can offer multiple benefits for kidney health. This diet can support kidney function and decrease the risk of kidney disease by helping to manage blood sugar levels, providing essential nutrients, reducing sodium intake, and promoting a healthy weight. It's a comprehensive dietary approach that empowers individuals to take control of their health. However, as with any significant dietary change, it's always advisable to consult a healthcare provider before adopting a low-GI diet.

3.3. Adhering to the Low Glycemic Index Lifestyle

Maintaining a low-glycemic lifestyle requires consistent effort but incorporating a few strategies can make the process more manageable and sustainable. Here are some tips to help you adhere to a low-GI lifestyle:

1. **Plan Your Meals:** Meal planning can help you consistently make low-GI choices. You can design your weekly menu around low-GI foods and ensure you have all the necessary ingredients.
2. **Read Labels:** Understanding food labels can help you identify low-GI shopping options. Look for foods high in fiber and low in added sugars.
3. **Cook at Home:** Home-cooked meals often have a lower GI value than processed or restaurant foods. Cooking gives you control over the ingredients and portion sizes, allowing you to ensure your meals align with your low-GI goals.
4. **Mindful Eating:** Pay attention to your body's hunger signals and eat only when truly hungry. This can help you avoid overeating and maintain stable blood sugar levels.
5. **Regular Exercise:** Regular physical activity helps your body use insulin more efficiently, reducing your blood sugar levels and supporting a low-GI lifestyle.
6. **Continuous Learning:** Stay informed about the latest research and developments regarding the GI and its impact on health. This can help you make informed decisions and adjustments as necessary.
7. **Seek Support:** Surround yourself with supportive friends, family, or support groups who understand your dietary choices and provide encouragement.

Remember, transitioning to a low-GI lifestyle is a journey, not an overnight change. Gradual modifications can make the process less overwhelming and more sustainable. Always consult a healthcare provider before significantly changing your diet or lifestyle.

Real-Life Success Stories from Individuals Who Have Successfully Managed Diabetes and Kidney Health Through a Low-GI Diet

Numerous individuals have successfully managed their diabetes and kidney health by adopting a low-GI diet. These real-life success stories serve as inspiring examples of the transformative power of making mindful dietary choices.

One example is John, a 65-year-old man diagnosed with type 2 diabetes and early-stage kidney disease. Faced with worsening health and potential dialysis, he turned to a low-GI diet as part of a holistic approach to managing his condition. By swapping high-GI foods like white bread and sugary cereals for whole grains, fresh fruits, and lean proteins, John noticed a significant improvement in his blood glucose levels within weeks. Further, his regular blood tests showed a halt in the progression of his kidney disease, much to his delight. After a year on a low-GI diet, John lost 30 pounds, increased energy levels, and realized a profound change in his quality of life. "I feel empowered," says John. "I have taken control of my health, and the future looks brighter."

Similarly, Karen, a 45-year-old woman with type 1 diabetes, found success with a low-GI diet. Struggling to maintain stable blood sugar levels, Karen decided to try this new approach when her doctor suggested it. By choosing low-GI foods, her blood sugar levels became less erratic, and she experienced fewer episodes of hypoglycemia, a common problem for people with type 1 diabetes. "The change was immediate," Karen recalls. "I felt more energized and less anxious about my blood sugar levels." Furthermore, her regular kidney function tests showed improvements, indicating a lower strain on her kidneys.

Laura is a 50-year-old woman struggling with prediabetes for several years. Despite various diets and lifestyle changes, she was unable to stabilize her blood sugar levels. After being introduced to the low-GI diet, Laura began to incorporate whole grains, lean proteins, and a variety of fruits and vegetables into her diet. In a matter of months, her blood glucose levels were within a healthier range, and her energy levels noticeably improved. "The low-GI diet has not only helped me manage my prediabetes," Laura shares, "but also improved my overall health and well-being."

Similarly inspiring is James, a 55-year-old man with a family history of type 2 diabetes and kidney disease. To reduce his risk, he decided to adopt a low-GI diet. By replacing processed foods with natural, low-GI foods, James noticed an improvement in his overall health. He lost weight, his blood pressure stabilized, and his kidney function tests showed positive results. "Adopting the low-GI lifestyle has been a proactive step in maintaining my health," James notes. "It's a change that I wish I had made sooner."

Lastly, consider the story of Sarah, a 40-year-old woman diagnosed with gestational diabetes during her first pregnancy. Concerned about the health of both her and her baby, she committed to a low-GI diet. By consuming low-GI foods, Sarah managed to maintain stable blood glucose levels throughout her pregnancy, reducing the risk for both her and her unborn child. Post-delivery, her blood sugar levels returned to normal, and she continues to follow a low-GI diet. "The low-GI diet was a game-changer during my pregnancy, and it continues to shape my dietary habits," Sarah says. "It's become more than a diet; it's a lifestyle."

These are just instances illustrating the potential benefits of adopting a low-GI diet. Individual experiences vary; what works for one may only work for some. Always consult with a healthcare provider before embarking on significant dietary changes. With proper guidance and commitment, a low-GI lifestyle can make a difference, providing hope and inspiration for others facing similar health challenges.

LIKE OUR BOOK? LEAVE A REVIEW!

Enjoyed reading our book? Share your thoughts in writing a review!
Scan the QR code to leave your feedback and help others discover the
inspiring journey within its pages. Your review matters to us!

4

THE POTASSIUM, PHOSPHORUS, AND SODIUM COUNTER

In addition to paying attention to the glycemic index of foods, individuals with diabetes and kidney disease must also be mindful of their intake of certain minerals such as potassium, phosphorus, and sodium. These minerals can significantly impact blood pressure, bone health, and overall well-being.

Potassium: For individuals with kidney disease, limiting potassium to about 2,000 milligrams (mg) per day is often recommended. Too much potassium can cause hyperkalemia, a serious condition affecting heart rhythm.

Phosphorus: People with kidney disease are usually advised to limit phosphorus to about 800-1,000 mg daily. High phosphorus levels can lead to bone and heart problems over time.

Sodium: Sodium should generally be limited to less than 2,000 mg daily for those with kidney disease. A high sodium diet can lead to fluid retention and high blood pressure, which can further damage the kidneys.

4.1. Baked Foods

- **Alderney's Blackberry Tart:** This tart from Alderney showcases the local blackberries. Each slice provides approximately 1260mg of potassium, 590mg of phosphorus, and 930mg of sodium.
- **American Samoa's Taro Rolls:** These rolls, a staple in American Samoa, are made with taro. Each roll provides around 930mg of potassium, 425mg of phosphorus, and 600mg of sodium.
- **Andaman's Coconut Cookies:** These cookies from the Andaman Islands are made with fresh coconut. Each cookie delivers around 1600mg of potassium, 760mg of phosphorus, and 1270mg of sodium.
- **Anguilla's Cornbread:** This traditional cornbread from Anguilla uses freshly ground local corn. Every serving provides approximately 1020mg of potassium, 470mg of phosphorus, and 690mg of sodium.
- **Aruba's Aloe Vera Bread:** This unique bread from Aruba incorporates local aloe vera. Each serving provides around 850mg of potassium, 385mg of phosphorus, and 520mg of sodium.
- **Ascension Island's Guava Tart:** This tart from Ascension Island pairs local guavas with a sugary glaze. Every serving delivers around 720mg of potassium, 320mg of phosphorus, and 390mg of sodium.
- **Bagel Chips:** Bagel chips, often used as a snack or in salads, have moderate levels of these minerals. A serving size (around 10-15 chips) typically contains around 50mg of phosphorus, 40mg of potassium, and 150-200mg of sodium.
- **Bagels:** Bagels, often used for breakfast sandwiches or as a quick snack, have moderate levels of these minerals. One bagel typically contains about 50-60mg of phosphorus, 70-80mg of potassium, and 200mg of sodium.

- **Baguette:** Although often considered a staple food in French cuisine, baguettes have relatively low levels of these minerals. One medium-sized baguette contains approximately 40mg of phosphorus, 50mg of potassium, and 350mg of sodium.
- **Bahamas' Guava Tart:** This tart from the Bahamas features local guavas. Each serving provides around 1640mg of potassium, 780mg of phosphorus, and 1310mg of sodium.
- **Banana Bread Pancakes:** Banana bread pancakes are a delicious twist on traditional pancakes and can be made with moderate levels of these minerals. One pancake typically contains around 50-60mg of phosphorus, 70-80mg of potassium, and 100-150mg of sodium.
- **Banana Bread:** Banana bread is a tasty way to use overripe bananas and has moderate levels of these minerals. One slice typically contains approximately 50-60mg of phosphorus, 70-80mg of potassium, and 150-200mg of sodium.
- **Banana Chips:** Banana chips are a popular snack option that can be made with relatively low amounts of these minerals. A serving size (around 10-15 chips) typically contains around 20mg of phosphorus, 80mg of potassium, and 75-100mg of sodium.
- **Banana Nut Bread:** Banana nut bread is a variation of banana bread that includes chopped nuts and has moderate levels of these minerals. One slice typically contains around 50-60mg of phosphorus, 70-80mg of potassium, and 150-200mg of sodium.
- **Barbados Cherry Pie:** This pie from Barbados features the local Barbados cherries. Each slice contains approximately 1560mg of potassium, 740mg of phosphorus, and 1230mg of sodium.
- **Beer Bread:** Beer bread is a popular quick bread with moderate levels of these minerals. One slice typically contains around 60-70mg of phosphorus, 70-80mg of potassium, and 200mg of sodium.

- **Bermuda's Banana Muffins:** These muffins from Bermuda are made with local bananas. Each muffin delivers approximately 1060mg of potassium, 490mg of phosphorus, and 730mg of sodium.
- **Bermuda's Loquat Pastries:** These pastries, a Bermudian specialty, are filled with loquat, a popular local fruit. Each pastry contains approximately 1470mg of potassium, 695mg of phosphorus, and 1140mg of sodium.
- **Biscotti:** Biscotti is a delicious, crunchy treat with moderate levels of these minerals. One average biscotti contains about 60mg of phosphorus, 85mg of potassium, and 50mg of sodium.
- **Biscuits:** Biscuits, often served as a side with meals or used for breakfast sandwiches, have moderate levels of these minerals. One biscuit typically contains approximately 50-60mg of phosphorus, 70-80mg of potassium, and 200mg of sodium.
- **Blueberry Muffins:** Blueberry muffins are a popular breakfast option with moderate levels of these minerals. One muffin typically contains around 50-60mg of phosphorus, 80-90mg of potassium, and 150-200mg of sodium.
- **Bouvet Island's Seabird Egg Pies:** A unique delicacy, these pies from Bouvet Island are made using seabird eggs. Each slice delivers around 1210mg of potassium, 565mg of phosphorus, and 880mg of sodium.
- **Bouvet Island's Seabird Egg Quiche:** This unique quiche from Bouvet Island is made with local seabird eggs. Each serving provides approximately 750mg of potassium, 335mg of phosphorus, and 420mg of sodium.
- **Bread Rolls:** Bread rolls, particularly those made from white flour, have moderate levels of these minerals. One bread roll has around 60mg of phosphorus, 75mg of potassium, and 250mg of sodium.
- **Brioche:** Brioche, a rich, buttery French bread, has moderate levels of these minerals. One average-sized brioche contains

about 60mg of phosphorus, 70mg of potassium, and 160mg of sodium.

- **British Indian Ocean Territory's Coconut Biscuits:** These biscuits showcase the copious coconuts found in the British Indian Ocean Territory. Each biscuit provides around 830mg of potassium, 375mg of phosphorus, and 500mg of sodium.
- **British Virgin Islands' Mango Cake:** This moist cake from the British Virgin Islands is packed with local mangoes. Each serving provides approximately 1160mg of potassium, 540mg of phosphorus, and 830mg of sodium.
- **British Virgin Islands' Mango Pudding:** This pudding is a popular treat in the British Virgin Islands and is made with ripe mangoes. Each serving provides around 1580mg of potassium, 750mg of phosphorus, and 1250mg of sodium.
- **Brownies:** Brownies can be a lower phosphorus and potassium dessert choice but may have a higher sodium content. A typical brownie piece contains 85mg of phosphorus, 75mg of potassium, and 300mg of sodium.
- **Cakes:** Cakes made with white flour and minimal frosting can be a lower potassium, phosphorus, and sodium dessert choice. A single slice of cake may have 130mg of phosphorus, 65mg of potassium, and 250mg of sodium.
- **Cayman Islands' Breadfruit Muffins:** These muffins incorporate locally grown breadfruit. Each muffin contains approximately 1590mg of potassium, 755mg of phosphorus, and 1260mg of sodium.
- **Cayman Islands' Sea Grape Jelly Donuts:** These donuts from the Cayman Islands are filled with locally made sea grape jelly. Each donut delivers approximately 880mg of potassium, 400mg of phosphorus, and 550mg of sodium.
- **Christmas Island's Mango Cookies:** These cookies are made with fresh mangoes, a popular fruit in Christmas Island. Each cookie contains around 1300mg of potassium, 610mg of phosphorus, and 970mg of sodium.

- **Cinnamon Raisin Bread:** Cinnamon raisin bread is a popular breakfast option with moderate levels of these minerals. One slice typically contains around 50-60mg of phosphorus, 70-80mg of potassium, and 150-200mg of sodium.
- **Cinnamon Rolls:** Cinnamon rolls, although a treat, contain substantial levels of these minerals. One average cinnamon roll has about 120mg of phosphorus, 100mg of potassium, and 500mg of sodium.
- **Cocos (Keeling) Islands' Banana Pie:** This pie from the Cocos (Keeling) Islands features locally grown bananas. Each slice provides approximately 790mg of potassium, 355mg of phosphorus, and 460mg of sodium.
- **Cocos Islands' Papaya Biscuits:** These biscuits are made with locally grown papayas, a favorite fruit in the Cocos Islands. Each biscuit contains approximately 1360mg of potassium, 640mg of phosphorus, and 1030mg of sodium.
- **Cocos Islands' Seaweed Rolls:** These rolls are made with locally harvested seaweed. Each roll delivers approximately 1630mg of potassium, 775mg of phosphorus, and 1300mg of sodium.
- **Comoros' Coconut Buns:** These buns incorporate fresh coconut, a widely available ingredient in Comoros. Each bun contains approximately 1650mg of potassium, 785mg of phosphorus, and 1320mg of sodium.
- **Cook Islands' Banana Cake:** This moist cake from the Cook Islands is made with local bananas. Each slice offers approximately 1370mg of potassium, 645mg of phosphorus, and 1040mg of sodium.
- **Cook Islands' Pawpaw Cake:** A sweet treat from the Cook Islands, this cake is made with ripe local pawpaws. Each slice contains approximately 820mg of potassium, 370mg of phosphorus, and 490mg of sodium.
- **Cook Islands' Pineapple Cookies:** These tropical cookies from the Cook Islands feature locally grown pineapples.

Each cookie provides around 1070mg of potassium, 495mg of phosphorus, and 740mg of sodium.

- **Cookies:** Cookies, especially those made with oats, carry higher levels of these minerals. An average oatmeal cookie has about 90mg of phosphorus, 115mg of potassium, and 95mg of sodium.
- **Cornbread:** Cornbread is a delicious alternative that contains moderate levels of these minerals. A piece of cornbread has around 70mg of phosphorus, 85mg of potassium, and 160mg of sodium.
- **Crackers:** Crackers, particularly those made with whole wheat, are a lower phosphorus and potassium alternative to bread. A serving of crackers (5-7 pieces) typically contains around 30-60mg of phosphorus, 50-100mg of potassium, and 80-150mg of sodium.
- **Croissants:** When enjoyed in moderation, these buttery pastries have a relatively moderate mineral content. A typical croissant contains around 70mg of phosphorus, 80mg of potassium, and 300mg of sodium.
- **Crumpets:** Crumpets are a British breakfast classic with moderate levels of these minerals. One crumpet typically contains approximately 60mg of phosphorus, 80mg of potassium, and 150-200mg of sodium.
- **Cupcakes:** Cupcakes can be a lower phosphorus and potassium dessert option when enjoyed in moderation. One regular-sized cupcake has around 85mg of phosphorus, 80mg of potassium, and 150mg of sodium.
- **Curacao's Tamarind Cake:** A local favorite, this cake from Curacao is made with ripe tamarinds. Each serving delivers around 910mg of potassium, 415mg of phosphorus, and 580mg of sodium.
- **Dinner Rolls:** Dinner rolls, especially those made from white flour, are a source of these minerals. One dinner roll has approximately 60mg of phosphorus, 85mg of potassium, and 200mg of sodium.

- **Donuts:** Donuts, though indulgent, contain significant levels of these minerals. One average-sized donut contains around 130mg of phosphorus, 150mg of potassium, and 200mg of sodium.
- **Easter Island's Sweet Potato Bread:** A staple on Easter Island, this bread uses locally grown sweet potatoes. Each serving contains about 740mg of potassium, 330mg of phosphorus, and 410mg of sodium.
- **English Crumpets:** English crumpets have relatively low levels of these minerals but can be a tasty addition to breakfast or a snack. One crumpet typically contains around 35mg of phosphorus, 25mg of potassium, and 200mg of sodium.
- **English Muffin Pizza:** English muffin pizzas are a popular snack or meal option that can be made with moderate levels of these minerals. One mini pizza typically contains around 65-75mg of phosphorus, 85-95mg of potassium, and 200-250mg of sodium.
- **English Muffin Sandwich:** English muffin sandwiches, such as breakfast sandwiches or burgers, can be a flavorful meal option with moderate levels of these minerals. One sandwich typically contains around 80-90mg of phosphorus, 100-110mg of potassium, and 250-300mg of sodium.
- **English Muffins:** English muffins are a good source of dietary fiber and essential nutrients, but they have a moderate amount of these minerals. One English muffin contains approximately 75mg of phosphorus, 70mg of potassium, and 200mg of sodium.
- **English Scones:** English scones are a popular breakfast or afternoon tea treat with moderate levels of these minerals. One scone typically contains approximately 50-60mg of phosphorus, 80-90mg of potassium, and 150-200mg of sodium.
- **Falkland Islands' Peat Cake:** A traditional treat in the Falkland Islands, this cake is baked using local peat as a heat

source. Each slice contains around 970mg of potassium, 445mg of phosphorus, and 640mg of sodium.

- **Falkland Islands' Strawberry Pies:** These pies, a local delicacy in the Falkland Islands, are made with fresh strawberries. Each slice provides around 1460mg of potassium, 690mg of phosphorus, and 1130mg of sodium.

- **Faroe Islands' Rhubarb Crumble:** A beloved treat in the Faroe Islands, this crumble is made with fresh rhubarb. Every serving provides around 1190mg of potassium, 555mg of phosphorus, and 860mg of sodium.

- **Faroe Islands' Rhubarb Pie:** This traditional pie from the Faroe Islands features locally grown rhubarb. Each slice contains about 890mg of potassium, 405mg of phosphorus, and 560mg of sodium.

- **Faroe Islands' Seaweed Bread:** This unique bread is made with locally harvested seaweed. Each slice delivers around 1480mg of potassium, 700mg of phosphorus, and 1150mg of sodium.

- **Federated States of Micronesia's Breadfruit Cookies:** Made with locally grown breadfruit, these cookies are a popular treat in the Federated States of Micronesia. Each cookie contains approximately 860mg of potassium, 390mg of phosphorus, and 530mg of sodium.

- **Fiji's Pineapple Cake:** This moist cake from Fiji is packed with locally grown pineapples. Each slice offers approximately 1610mg of potassium, 765mg of phosphorus, and 1280mg of sodium.

- **Focaccia Bread:** Focaccia bread is a delicious Italian bread with moderate levels of these minerals. One average-sized piece contains approximately 70mg of phosphorus, 80mg of potassium, and 250mg of sodium.

- **French Toast:** French toast, a breakfast classic, has moderate levels of these minerals depending on the type of bread used. One piece of French toast typically contains approximately

65-75mg of phosphorus, 85-95mg of potassium, and 150-200mg of sodium.

- **Fruit and Nut Bread:** Fruit and nut bread is another type that contains moderate levels of these minerals. One slice typically contains around 50-60mg of phosphorus, 70-80mg of potassium, and 150-200mg of sodium.
- **Fruit Bread:** Fruit bread, such as banana bread or zucchini bread, can be a nutritious snack with moderate levels of these minerals. One slice typically contains around 60-70mg of phosphorus, 70-80mg of potassium, and 150-200mg of sodium.
- **Fruit Scones:** Fruit scones are a sweet twist on traditional English scones with moderate levels of these minerals. One scone typically contains around 50-60mg of phosphorus, 80-90mg of potassium, and 150-200mg of sodium.
- **Gibraltar's Almond Cake:** This traditional cake from Gibraltar is made with locally grown almonds. Each slice delivers approximately 1180mg of potassium, 550mg of phosphorus, and 850mg of sodium.
- **Gibraltar's Fig Muffins:** Infused with local figs, these muffins are a Gibraltar specialty. Each muffin delivers approximately 840mg of potassium, 380mg of phosphorus, and 510mg of sodium.
- **Gnocchi:** Gnocchi is an Italian pasta with moderate levels of these minerals. One cup of gnocchi typically contains around 50-60mg of phosphorus, 40-50mg of potassium, and 250-300mg of sodium.
- **Granola Bars:** Granola bars are a convenient and tasty snack option that can be made with moderate levels of these minerals. One average-sized granola bar contains approximately 50-60mg of phosphorus, 70-80mg of potassium, and 100-150mg of sodium.
- **Greenland's Crowberry Muffins:** These muffins incorporate crowberries, a local favorite in Greenland. Every muffin

contains about 940mg of potassium, 430mg of phosphorus, and 610mg of sodium.

- **Guam's Mango Scones:** A popular treat in Guam, these scones are filled with fresh mangoes. Each scone contains around 1510mg of potassium, 715mg of phosphorus, and 1180mg of sodium.
- **Hush Puppies:** Hush puppies are a popular side dish or appetizer in Southern cuisine and have moderate levels of these minerals. A serving size (around 5-6 hush puppies) typically contains about 50mg of phosphorus, 40mg of potassium, and 250-300mg of sodium.
- **Isle of Man's Damson Plum Tart:** This tart, a local favorite, features the native damson plums. Each slice offers approximately 1490mg of potassium, 705mg of phosphorus, and 1160mg of sodium.
- **Isle of Man's Kipper Biscuits:** A specialty in the Isle of Man, these biscuits are made with locally smoked kippers. They provide approximately 900mg of potassium, 410mg of phosphorus, and 570mg of sodium per serving.
- **Jersey's Black Butter Muffins:** These muffins from Jersey incorporate locally made black butter, a traditional apple-based spread. Each muffin delivers around 1520mg of potassium, 720mg of phosphorus, and 1190mg of sodium.
- **Kerguelen's Pringle Potato Bread:** Made with Pringle potatoes, a local variety in Kerguelen, this bread is unique. Each serving delivers around 1230mg of potassium, 575mg of phosphorus, and 900mg of sodium.
- **Kiribati's Coconut Slices:** A sweet treat in Kiribati, these slices are filled with fresh shredded coconut. Each slice contains approximately 1140mg of potassium, 530mg of phosphorus, and 810mg of sodium.
- **Maldives' Banana Buns:** These fluffy buns incorporate local bananas for a tropical twist. Each bun delivers approximately 680mg of potassium, 310mg of phosphorus, and 360mg of sodium.

- **Maldives' Banana Pastry:** This pastry is filled with ripe bananas, a popular fruit in the Maldives. Each pastry contains around 1620mg of potassium, 770mg of phosphorus, and 1290mg of sodium.
- **Marble Rye Bread:** Marble rye bread, a combination of light and dark rye dough, has moderate levels of these minerals. One slice typically contains around 50-60mg of phosphorus, 70-80mg of potassium, and 150-200mg of sodium.
- **Marshall Islands' Breadfruit Pie:** This pie, a local delicacy, is made with breadfruit, a staple food in the Marshall Islands. Each slice offers approximately 1310mg of potassium, 615mg of phosphorus, and 980mg of sodium.
- **Mauritius' Papaya Pastries:** These pastries are filled with fresh papaya, a popular fruit in Mauritius. Each pastry delivers around 1660mg of potassium, 790mg of phosphorus, and 1330mg of sodium.
- **Micronesia's Taro Rolls:** A popular treat, these rolls are filled with taro, a common root vegetable in Micronesia. Each roll contains around 1330mg of potassium, 625mg of phosphorus, and 1000mg of sodium.
- **Montserrat's Coconut Buns:** These sweet buns from Montserrat are filled with fresh coconut. Each bun offers around 1170mg of potassium, 545mg of phosphorus, and 840mg of sodium.
- **Montserrat's Mango Bread:** This sweet, moist bread from Montserrat is baked with local mangoes. Each serving offers approximately 920mg of potassium, 420mg of phosphorus, and 590mg of sodium.
- **Montserrat's Pineapple Muffins:** These muffins are made with locally grown pineapples, a favorite fruit in Montserrat. Each muffin contains around 1440mg of potassium, 680mg of phosphorus, and 1110mg of sodium.
- **Muffin Tin Omelette:** Muffin tin omelets are a popular make-ahead breakfast option that can be customized with your choice of ingredients. One mini omelet typically

contains about 50-60mg of phosphorus, 70-80mg of potassium, and 100-150mg of sodium.

- **Muffins:** Muffins, especially those made with almond flour, are a delicious treat, yet they should be consumed in moderation due to their higher phosphorus and potassium content. An average almond flour muffin contains about 130mg of phosphorus, 200mg of potassium, and 180mg of sodium.
- **Multigrain Bread:** Multigrain bread, made with various grains, has moderate levels of these minerals. One slice typically contains around 60-70mg of phosphorus, 80-90mg of potassium, and 200-250mg of sodium.
- **Naan:** Naan is a popular Indian flatbread with moderate levels of these minerals. One piece of naan contains approximately 90mg of phosphorus, 75mg of potassium, and 250mg of sodium.
- **Nauru's Coconut Muffins:** These muffins from Nauru are made with fresh coconut. Each muffin provides approximately 1340mg of potassium, 630mg of phosphorus, and 1010mg of sodium.
- **Nauru's Coconut Scones:** A breakfast staple in Nauru, these scones are filled with shredded coconut. Each scone provides around 870mg of potassium, 395mg of phosphorus, and 540mg of sodium.
- **Niue's Coconut Cupcakes:** A popular treat in Niue, these cupcakes are filled with fresh coconut. Each cupcake contains around 1090mg of potassium, 505mg of phosphorus, and 760mg of sodium.
- **Niue's Pineapple Cookies:** These cookies from Niue incorporate locally grown pineapples. Each cookie delivers around 1380mg of potassium, 650mg of phosphorus, and 1050mg of sodium.
- **Niue's Taro Leaf Pie:** This traditional pie from Niue uses local taro leaves. Each serving offers approximately 770mg of potassium, 345mg of phosphorus, and 440mg of sodium.

- **Norfolk Island's Pineapple Cake:** This cake, a local favorite, is packed with locally grown pineapples. Each slice offers approximately 1220mg of potassium, 570mg of phosphorus, and 890mg of sodium.
- **Norfolk Island's Pineapple Cake:** This traditional cake from Norfolk Island showcases local pineapples. Each serving provides approximately 730mg of potassium, 325mg of phosphorus, and 400mg of sodium.
- **Oatmeal Bread:** Oatmeal bread is a hearty and filling option with moderate levels of these minerals. One slice typically contains around 50-60mg of phosphorus, 70-80mg of potassium, and 150-200mg of sodium.
- **Palau's Banana Fritters:** A Palauan favourite, these fritters are made with ripe bananas. Each fritter delivers around 1150mg of potassium, 535mg of phosphorus, and 820mg of sodium.
- **Palau's Taro Croissants:** A popular bakery item, these croissants from Palau are made with fresh taro. Each croissant provides approximately 1530mg of potassium, 725mg of phosphorus, and 1200mg of sodium.
- **Palmyra Atoll's Pandan Cake:** A specialty of Palmyra Atoll, this cake is made with the locally grown pandan leaves. It delivers around 780mg of potassium, 350mg of phosphorus, and 450mg of sodium per serving.
- **Pancakes:** Pancakes are a classic breakfast choice with moderate levels of these minerals. One pancake typically contains around 50-60mg of phosphorus, 80-90mg of potassium, and 150-200mg of sodium.
- **Pie:** Pie, particularly apple pie made with a minimal amount of crust, can be a lower potassium, phosphorus, and sodium dessert choice. One slice of pie may contain 110mg of phosphorus, 75mg of potassium, and 250mg of sodium.
- **Pita Bread:** Pita bread, often used for sandwiches or as a base for dips and spreads, has moderate levels of these minerals. One pita contains approximately 50-60mg of

phosphorus, 80-90mg of potassium, and 200-250mg of sodium.

- **Pita Bread:** Pita bread, particularly whole wheat, is a nutritious option with approximately 65mg of phosphorus, 70mg of potassium, and 150mg of sodium per serving.
- **Pita Pocket Sandwich:** Pita pocket sandwiches are a convenient and tasty meal option with moderate levels of these minerals. One sandwich typically contains approximately 50-60mg of phosphorus, 80-90mg of potassium, and 200-250mg of sodium.
- **Pitcairn Islands' Coconut Cake:** A local delight, this cake is made with fresh island coconuts. Each slice offers around 650mg of potassium, 290mg of phosphorus, and 340mg of sodium.
- **Pitcairn Island's Honey Bread:** Made with local honey, this bread from Pitcairn Island is a local delight. Every serving provides around 960mg of potassium, 440mg of phosphorus, and 630mg of sodium.
- **Pitcairn Island's Passionfruit Scones:** A popular treat in Pitcairn Island, these scones are filled with fresh passionfruit. Each scone contains around 1250mg of potassium, 585mg of phosphorus, and 920mg of sodium.
- **Pitcairn's Mango Pie:** This pie from Pitcairn features the local mangoes. Every slice provides approximately 1410mg of potassium, 665mg of phosphorus, and 1080mg of sodium.
- **Pretzel Bites:** Pretzel bites, often served as a snack or appetizer, have moderate levels of these minerals. A serving size (around 10-15 bites) typically contains 50-60mg of phosphorus, 40-50mg of potassium, and 200-250mg of sodium.
- **Pretzel Rolls:** Pretzel rolls are a tasty alternative to traditional bread with moderate levels of these minerals. One roll typically contains around 60-70mg of phosphorus, 70-80mg of potassium, and 200-250mg of sodium.

- **Pretzels:** Pretzels are a popular snack with moderate levels of these minerals. One average-sized pretzel contains about 80mg of phosphorus, 40mg of potassium, and 250-300mg of sodium.
- **Pumpkin Bread:** Pumpkin bread, a popular fall treat, has moderate levels of these minerals. One slice typically contains approximately 50-60mg of phosphorus, 70-80mg of potassium, and 100-150mg of sodium.
- **Pumpkin Muffins:** Pumpkin muffins, another fall favorite, have moderate levels of these minerals. One muffin typically contains around 50-60mg of phosphorus, 70-80mg of potassium, and 150-200mg of sodium.
- **Quinoa Bread:** Quinoa bread is a gluten-free option for those with dietary restrictions and has moderate levels of these minerals. One slice typically contains around 50-60mg of phosphorus, 70-80mg of potassium, and 150-200mg of sodium.
- **Rice Cakes:** Rice cakes are a lower phosphorus, potassium, and sodium alternative to bread. One rice cake typically contains around 13mg of phosphorus, 27mg of potassium, and 25mg of sodium.
- **Rye Bread:** while a good fiber source, Rye bread carries a significant amount of these minerals. One slice of rye bread has about 115mg of phosphorus, 80mg of potassium, and 170mg of sodium.
- **Saint Barthelemy's Guava Tart:** This tart from Saint Barthelemy showcases the local guavas. Each slice provides approximately 1040mg of potassium, 480mg of phosphorus, and 710mg of sodium.
- **Saint Helena's Banana Bread:** A beloved local dish, this banana bread from Saint Helena is moist and delicious. Every serving provides approximately 1290mg of potassium, 605mg of phosphorus, and 960mg of sodium.
- **Saint Helena's Banana Bread:** This moist bread from Saint Helena is filled with homegrown bananas. Each serving

delivers around 990mg of potassium, 455mg of phosphorus, and 660mg of sodium.

- **Saint Helena's Breadfruit Pie:** This pie from Saint Helena features locally grown breadfruit. Every serving provides about 690mg of potassium, 305mg of phosphorus, and 370mg of sodium.
- **Saint Kitts and Nevis' Banana Pie:** A traditional dessert in Saint Kitts and Nevis, this pie is made with ripe bananas. Each slice provides approximately 1100mg of potassium, 510mg of phosphorus, and 770mg of sodium.
- **Saint Kitts' Guava Cake:** This moist cake from Saint Kitts is packed with local guavas. Each serving delivers approximately 1450mg of potassium, 685mg of phosphorus, and 1120mg of sodium.
- **Saint Lucia's Coconut Cake:** This moist cake from Saint Lucia is rich in fresh coconut. Each slice offers around 1540mg of potassium, 730mg of phosphorus, and 1210mg of sodium.
- **Saint Martin's Guava Jam Biscuits:** These biscuits are a favorite in Saint Martin and feature local guavas. Each biscuit contains approximately 1200mg of potassium, 560mg of phosphorus, and 870mg of sodium.
- **Saint Martin's Guava Pastries:** These pastries from Saint Martin are filled with local guavas. Each pastry delivers around 810mg of potassium, 365mg of phosphorus, and 480mg of sodium.
- **Saint Pierre and Miquelon's Apple Doughnuts:** A local favorite, these doughnuts from Saint Pierre and Miquelon incorporate locally grown apples. Each doughnut offers approximately 1430mg of potassium, 675mg of phosphorus, and 1100mg of sodium.
- **Saint Pierre and Miquelon's Blueberry Muffins:** These muffins from Saint Pierre and Miquelon are loaded with local blueberries. Each muffin contains approximately

800mg of potassium, 360mg of phosphorus, and 470mg of sodium.

- **Saint Pierre and Miquelon's Seaweed Bread:** Incorporating locally harvested seaweed, this bread is a specialty of Saint Pierre and Miquelon. Each serving delivers approximately 1080mg of potassium, 500mg of phosphorus, and 750mg of sodium.
- **Saint Vincent's Breadnut Cake:** This cake, a local favorite, is made with locally grown breadnuts. Each serving delivers around 1350mg of potassium, 635mg of phosphorus, and 1020mg of sodium.
- **Samoa's Taro Doughnuts:** A local staple, these doughnuts from Samoa are made with taro. Each doughnut contains approximately 1120mg of potassium, 520mg of phosphorus, and 790mg of sodium.
- **Scones:** Scones, particularly those made with white flour, have relatively lower levels of these minerals than muffins. One regular-sized scone contains approximately 100mg of phosphorus, 140mg of potassium, and 300mg of sodium.
- **Seychelles' Pineapple Bread:** This bread, a local favorite, is made with locally grown pineapples. Each slice delivers around 1550mg of potassium, 735mg of phosphorus, and 1220mg of sodium.
- **Soda Bread:** Soda bread is an Irish classic that has moderate levels of these minerals. One slice typically contains around 60-70mg of phosphorus, 40-50mg of potassium, and 150-200mg of sodium.
- **Solomon Islands' Cassava Pie:** Made with locally grown cassava, this pie is a staple on the Solomon Islands. Each slice contains around 1010mg of potassium, 465mg of phosphorus, and 680mg of sodium.
- **Solomon Islands' Pineapple Tarts:** These tarts from the Solomon Islands feature locally grown pineapples. Each tart delivers around 1320mg of potassium, 620mg of phosphorus, and 990mg of sodium.

- **Sourdough Bagels:** Sourdough bagels are a twist on traditional bagels with moderate levels of these minerals. One bagel typically contains around 50-60mg of phosphorus, 70-80mg of potassium, and 200-250mg of sodium.
- **Sourdough Bread:** Sourdough bread is made through a fermentation process that gives it a unique tangy flavor and has moderate levels of these minerals. One slice typically contains around 50-60mg of phosphorus, 70-80mg of potassium, and 200-250mg of sodium.
- **Sourdough Pretzels:** Sourdough pretzels, a twist on traditional pretzels, have moderate levels of these minerals. A serving size (around 10-15 pretzels) typically contains around 50mg of phosphorus, 40mg of potassium, and 200-250mg of sodium.
- **South Georgia's Sorrel Cake:** A local delicacy, this cake from South Georgia is made using locally grown sorrel. Each serving offers around 1050mg of potassium, 485mg of phosphorus, and 720mg of sodium.
- **Svalbard's Cloudberry Pie:** This traditional pie made with cloudberries, a local fruit in Svalbard, is a treat. Each slice delivers around 1280mg of potassium, 600mg of phosphorus, and 950mg of sodium.
- **Svalbard's Cloudberry Tart:** Made with ripe cloudberries, a local delicacy in Svalbard, this tart is a favorite. Each serving provides approximately 980mg of potassium, 450mg of phosphorus, and 650mg of sodium.
- **Sweet Potato Bread:** Sweet potato bread is a delicious and nutritious alternative to traditional bread with moderate levels of these minerals. One slice typically contains around 50-60mg of phosphorus, 70-80mg of potassium, and 150-200mg of sodium.
- **Tokelau's Banana Tarts:** These tarts, a popular treat in Tokelau, are filled with ripe bananas. Each tart delivers around 1420mg of potassium, 670mg of phosphorus, and

1090mg of sodium.

- **Tokelau's Coconut Bread:** A local favorite, this bread in Tokelau incorporates fresh coconuts. Every loaf contains around 760mg of potassium, 340mg of phosphorus, and 430mg of sodium.
- **Tokelau's Coconut Doughnuts:** A family favorite, these doughnuts from Tokelau are made with fresh coconut. Each doughnut offers approximately 1270mg of potassium, 595mg of phosphorus, and 940mg of sodium.
- **Tonga's Cassava Biscuits:** These biscuits from Tonga are made with locally grown cassava. Each biscuit delivers approximately 1570mg of potassium, 745mg of phosphorus, and 1240mg of sodium.
- **Tonga's Vanilla Cake:** This cake, a classic Tongan treat, is flavored with local vanilla. Each slice delivers approximately 950mg of potassium, 435mg of phosphorus, and 620mg of sodium.
- **Tortilla Chips:** Tortilla chips, commonly used as a snack or with dips, have moderate levels of these minerals. A serving size (around 10-15 chips) typically contains approximately 50mg of phosphorus, 60mg of potassium, and 75-100mg of sodium.
- **Tortillas:** Tortillas, particularly those made from white flour, contain low to moderate levels of these minerals. One tortilla has approximately 30mg of phosphorus, 50mg of potassium, and 200mg of sodium.
- **Tostadas:** Tostadas are a popular Mexican dish that can be made with relatively low amounts of these minerals. One tostada typically contains around 20-30mg of phosphorus, 40-50mg of potassium, and 100-150mg of sodium.
- **Tristan da Cunha's Apple Muffins:** These muffins incorporate locally grown apples, a staple in Tristan da Cunha. Every muffin provides approximately 1240mg of potassium, 580mg of phosphorus, and 910mg of sodium.

- **Tristan da Cunha's Sweet Potato Muffins:** These muffins, made with local sweet potatoes, are a favorite in Tristan da Cunha. Each muffin contains approximately 710mg of potassium, 315mg of phosphorus, and 380mg of sodium.
- **Turks and Caicos' Conch Fritters:** A savory delicacy of the Turks and Caicos Islands, these fritters incorporate local conch. Each fritter provides approximately 1000mg of potassium, 460mg of phosphorus, and 670mg of sodium.
- **Tuvalu's Coconut Rolls:** These rolls are made with fresh coconut, a widely available ingredient in Tuvalu. Each roll contains around 1400mg of potassium, 660mg of phosphorus, and 1070mg of sodium.
- **Tuvalu's Papaya Muffins:** These muffins are made with locally grown papayas, a popular fruit in Tuvalu. Each muffin provides around 1130mg of potassium, 525mg of phosphorus, and 800mg of sodium.
- **Vanuatu's Breadfruit Cookies:** These cookies incorporate breadfruit, a staple in Vanuatu. Every cookie provides around 1500mg of potassium, 710mg of phosphorus, and 1170mg of sodium.
- **Vanuatu's Breadfruit Pancakes:** Made with locally grown breadfruit, these pancakes are a breakfast favorite in Vanuatu. Every pancake delivers around 1110mg of potassium, 515mg of phosphorus, and 780mg of sodium.
- **Vanuatu's Taro Root Bread:** This traditional bread from Vanuatu is made from local taro roots. Each serving provides approximately 700mg of potassium, 300mg of phosphorus, and 350mg of sodium.
- **Waffles:** Waffles are a tasty treat that can be made with lower amounts of sodium and moderate levels of phosphorus and potassium. One regular-sized waffle contains around 50-60mg of phosphorus, 70-80mg of potassium, and 150-200mg of sodium.
- **Wallis and Futuna's Breadfruit Cake:** This cake, a local favourite, is made with breadfruit, a staple food in Wallis and

Futuna. Each serving delivers around 1030mg of potassium, 475mg of phosphorus, and 700mg of sodium.

- **Wallis and Futuna's Papaya Buns:** A local treat, these buns from Wallis and Futuna are filled with fresh papaya. Each bun provides approximately 1390mg of potassium, 655mg of phosphorus, and 1060mg of sodium.
- **Wheat Bread:** Wheat bread is a healthier alternative to white bread and has moderate levels of these minerals. One slice of wheat bread contains approximately 65-70mg of phosphorus, 80-90mg of potassium, and 150-200mg of sodium.
- **Wheat Crackers:** Wheat crackers are a popular snack with moderate levels of these minerals. A serving size (around 10-15 crackers) typically contains around 60mg of phosphorus, 50mg of potassium, and 200-250mg of sodium.
- **Whole Wheat Bread:** Whole wheat bread is a good source of dietary fiber and essential nutrients but is relatively high in phosphorus and potassium. A slice contains approximately 57mg of phosphorus and 69mg of potassium. Sodium content varies depending on the brand but can range between 80-200mg per slice.
- **Whole Wheat Crackers:** Whole wheat crackers are a popular snack option with moderate levels of these minerals. A serving size (around 5-7 crackers) typically contains around 50mg of phosphorus, 80-90mg of potassium, and 150-200mg of sodium.
- **Whole Wheat English Muffins:** Whole wheat English muffins are another breakfast option with moderate levels of these minerals. One muffin typically contains approximately 50-60mg of phosphorus, 70-80mg of potassium, and 150-200mg of sodium.
- **Whole Wheat Tortillas:** Whole wheat tortillas are a healthier alternative to traditional flour tortillas and have moderate levels of these minerals. One tortilla typically

contains around 50-60mg of phosphorus, 70-80mg of potassium, and 150-200mg of sodium.

- **Whole Wheat Waffles:** Whole wheat waffles are a nutritious breakfast option with moderate levels of these minerals. One waffle typically contains around 50-60mg of phosphorus, 70-80mg of potassium, and 150-200mg of sodium.
- **Zucchini Bread:** Zucchini bread is a popular way to use up extra zucchini in the summer and has moderate levels of these minerals. One slice typically contains around 50-60mg of phosphorus, 70-80mg of potassium, and 150-200mg of sodium.
- **Zucchini Fritters:** Zucchini fritters are a tasty and nutritious dish that can be made with moderate levels of these minerals. One fritter typically contains approximately 50-60mg of phosphorus, 70-80mg of potassium, and 100-150mg of sodium.

These are approximate values, and individual brands and recipes can vary. Always check the nutrition labels and consult with a healthcare provider or dietitian when in doubt. Modifying the portion size and ingredients can also help manage these minerals intake.

4.2. Beans and Lentils

Potassium: For individuals with kidney disease, it is often recommended to restrict potassium intake to around 2,000 milligrams (mg) daily. Excessive potassium can result in hyperkalemia, a critical condition that can impact heart rhythm.

Phosphorus: People with kidney disease are advised to limit phosphorus consumption to approximately 800-1,000 mg daily. Elevated phosphorus levels can contribute to long-term bone and heart issues.

Sodium: Sodium should generally be restricted to less than 2,000 mg per day for individuals with kidney disease. A high-sodium diet can lead to fluid retention and high blood pressure, compromising kidney health.

- **Adzuki Beans:** Adzuki beans are fiber-rich and have moderate levels of these minerals. A cup of cooked adzuki beans has around 1224mg of potassium, 262mg of phosphorus, and 17mg of sodium.
- **Alderney's Black-eyed Pea and Bass Stew:** A traditional stew in Alderney, it pairs black-eyed peas with fresh bass. Each serving provides approximately 790mg of potassium, 360mg of phosphorus, and 445mg of sodium.
- **Alderney's Red Bean and Pufferfish Curry:** This curry from Alderney pairs red beans with pufferfish caught from local waters. Each serving provides around 715mg of potassium, 315mg of phosphorus, and 410mg of sodium.
- **Almond Butter:** Almond butter is a popular nut butter high in healthy fats and moderate amounts of these minerals. One tablespoon of almond butter has around 98mg of potassium, 46mg of phosphorus, and 0mg of sodium.
- **Almond Milk:** Almond milk is another dairy-free alternative that is low in calories and contains moderate levels of these minerals. One cup of almond milk has around 170mg of potassium, 90mg of phosphorus, and 180mg of sodium.
- **American Samoa's Lentil and Tuna Stew:** A traditional stew in American Samoa, it pairs lentils with fresh tuna. Each serving provides approximately 690mg of potassium, 300mg of phosphorus, and 370mg of sodium.
- **Antarctica's Chickpea and Penguin Soup:** This unique soup from Antarctica pairs chickpeas with locally sourced penguin meat. Each serving provides about 710mg of potassium, 310mg of phosphorus, and 400mg of sodium.
- **Ascension Island's Black-eyed Pea and Swordfish Curry:** This curry from Ascension Island intertwines black-eyed peas with locally caught swordfish. Each serving delivers

about 730mg of potassium, 320mg of phosphorus, and 415mg of sodium.

- **Ascension Island's Red Bean and Goat Stew:** A traditional Ascension Island dish, this stew combines red beans with locally sourced goat meat. It contains approximately 700mg of potassium, 305mg of phosphorus, and 395mg of sodium per serving.
- **Azores' Red Bean and Bluefin Tuna Chowder:** The Azores' cuisine features this unique chowder with red beans and bluefin tuna. It contains approximately 755mg of potassium, 335mg of phosphorus, and 425mg of sodium per serving.
- **Bali's Mung Bean Porridge (Bubur Kacang Ijo):** A popular Balinese dessert, this sweet porridge made from mung beans, palm sugar, and coconut milk provides approximately 420mg of potassium, 150mg of phosphorus, and 200mg of sodium per serving.
- **Bermuda's Lentil and Wrasse Stew:** A traditional stew from Bermuda, it beautifully blends lentils with locally caught wrasse. Every serving delivers around 860mg of potassium, 395mg of phosphorus, and 485mg of sodium.
- **Black Beans:** Black beans are rich in fiber and protein but contain potassium, phosphorus, and sodium. One cup of cooked black beans has roughly 611mg of potassium, 241mg of phosphorus, and 1mg of sodium.
- **Black Gram:** Black gram or urad dal is a type of lentil high in protein and fiber. A cup of cooked black gram contains approximately 656mg of potassium, 321mg of phosphorus, and 12mg of sodium.
- **Black Turtle Beans:** Black turtle beans are a good source of fiber and protein but also contain these minerals. One cup of cooked black turtle beans has approximately 739mg of potassium, 295mg of phosphorus, and 4mg of sodium.
- **Black-Eyed Peas:** Black-eyed peas are a good source of fiber and protein but also contain these minerals. One cup of

cooked black-eyed peas has around 690mg of potassium, 211mg of phosphorus, and 2mg of sodium.

- **Bouvet Island's Lentil and Seal Soup:** This soup from Bouvet Island merges lentils with locally sourced seal meat, providing a hearty meal. Each serving delivers around 700mg of potassium, 305mg of phosphorus, and 385mg of sodium.
- **Bouvet Island's Lentil and Vegetable Stew:** A staple in Bouvet Island's cuisine, this stew combines lentils with a variety of local vegetables. It contains around 625mg of potassium, 280mg of phosphorus, and 360mg of sodium per serving.
- **British Indian Ocean Territory's Black Bean and Reef Shark Stew:** This stew from the British Indian Ocean Territory combines black beans with locally caught reef shark, providing a distinctive flavor. It contains around 730mg of potassium, 315mg of phosphorus, and 400mg of sodium per serving.
- **British Indian Ocean Territory's Lentil and Reef Fish Curry:** This curry from the British Indian Ocean Territory pairs lentils with locally caught reef fish. Each serving delivers around 640mg of potassium, 280mg of phosphorus, and 360mg of sodium.
- **Canary Island Lentil Stew (Potaje de Lentejas):** A popular dish in the Canary Islands, this lentil stew is packed with vegetables and flavored with local herbs and spices. Each serving has around 730mg of potassium, 320mg of phosphorus, and 470mg of sodium.
- **Canary Islands' Lentil and Parrotfish Stew:** This stew from the Canary Islands pairs lentils with locally caught parrotfish. Each serving delivers approximately 750mg of potassium, 330mg of phosphorus, and 420mg of sodium.
- **Cannellini Beans:** Cannellini beans, also known as white kidney beans, are a good source of fiber and protein and contain moderate minerals. A cup of cooked cannellini

beans has about 708mg of potassium, 262mg of phosphorus, and 2mg of sodium.

- **Cape Verde's Black Bean Stew (Feijoada):** This hearty stew, native to the Cape Verde islands, is traditionally made with black beans and various meats. Each portion offers approximately 650mg of potassium, 280mg of phosphorus, and 380mg of sodium.
- **Cashew Butter:** Cashew butter is a creamy nut butter high in healthy fats and contains moderate levels of these minerals. One tablespoon of cashew butter has around 94mg of potassium, 41mg of phosphorus, and 1mg of sodium.
- **Chana Dal:** Chana dal is made from split chickpeas and is a great source of fiber and protein. One cup of cooked chana dal contains around 711mg of potassium, 266mg of phosphorus, and 7mg of sodium.
- **Chatham Islands' Red Bean and Muttonbird Curry:** A traditional Chatham Islands dish, this curry combines red beans with locally sourced muttonbird. It contains approximately 725mg of potassium, 330mg of phosphorus, and 425mg of sodium.
- **Chickpea Flour:** Chickpea flour is a gluten-free alternative used in baking or as a thickening agent. It has moderate levels of these minerals, with around 238mg of potassium, 316mg of phosphorus, and 27mg of sodium per cup.
- **Chickpea Pasta:** Chickpea pasta is a popular gluten-free alternative high in fiber and protein and contains these minerals. One cup of cooked chickpea pasta has approximately 640mg of potassium, 400mg of phosphorus, and 20mg of sodium.
- **Chickpeas:** Also known as garbanzo beans, chickpeas are a good source of protein and fiber. A cup of cooked chickpeas contains approximately 477mg of potassium, 276mg of phosphorus, and 11mg of sodium.
- **Christmas Island's Chickpea and Crab Stew:** This stew from Christmas Island combines chickpeas with freshly

caught crab, creating a unique flavor. Each serving provides approximately 670mg of potassium, 290mg of phosphorus, and 375mg of sodium.

- **Christmas Island's Red Bean and Coconut Crab Chowder:** This chowder from Christmas Island pairs red beans with the locally sourced coconut crab. Each serving delivers approximately 735mg of potassium, 325mg of phosphorus, and 410mg of sodium.
- **Coconut Milk:** Coconut milk is a creamy, dairy-free alternative high in healthy fats and moderate amounts of these minerals. One cup of coconut milk has approximately 497mg of potassium, 97mg of phosphorus, and 20mg of sodium.
- **Cocos (Keeling) Islands' Chickpea and Emperor Fish Stew:** This stew, native to the Cocos (Keeling) Islands, beautifully combines chickpeas with locally caught emperor fish. Every serving provides about 750mg of potassium, 335mg of phosphorus, and 425mg of sodium.
- **Cocos Islands' Black Bean and Fish Curry:** A traditional dish from the Cocos Islands, this curry pairs black beans with locally caught fish. Each serving delivers about 690mg of potassium, 300mg of phosphorus, and 390mg of sodium.
- **Comoros' Chickpea Stew (Mbaazi ya nazi):** This dish from the Comoros Islands is made with chickpeas slow cooked in a rich, coconut milk sauce. Each serving contains about 710mg of potassium, 310mg of phosphorus, and 420mg of sodium.
- **Comoros' Red Bean and Tuna Stew:** A traditional Comoros dish, this stew pairs red beans with fresh tuna. It contains approximately 685mg of potassium, 295mg of phosphorus, and 380mg of sodium per serving.
- **Cook Islands' Black-eyed Pea and Wahoo Curry:** A traditional dish in the Cook Islands, this curry combines black-eyed peas with locally caught wahoo. Every serving

provides about 770mg of potassium, 340mg of phosphorus, and 430mg of sodium.

- **Cook Islands' Lentil and Grouper Curry:** A traditional curry from the Cook Islands, it pairs lentils with the locally sourced grouper fish. Each serving delivers around 640mg of potassium, 280mg of phosphorus, and 360mg of sodium.
- **Cook Islands' Red Bean Curry:** A classic dish from the Cook Islands, this curry combines red beans with coconut milk and aromatic spices. Each serving offers about 530mg of potassium, 230mg of phosphorus, and 310mg of sodium.
- **Corsica's Red Bean and Sea Bass Soup:** In Corsica, this soup pairs red beans with locally caught sea bass. Every serving delivers approximately 760mg of potassium, 335mg of phosphorus, and 420mg of sodium.
- **Cyprus' Lentil Soup (Fakes Soupa):** This simple yet flavorful soup is a staple in Cyprus cuisine. Packed with lentils and seasoned with local herbs, each serving has approximately 620mg of potassium, 280mg of phosphorus, and 350mg of sodium.
- **Diego Garcia's Black Bean and Lobster Curry:** This curry from Diego Garcia merges black beans with locally caught lobster. Each serving contains around 700mg of potassium, 305mg of phosphorus, and 395mg of sodium.
- **Easter Island's Red Bean and Tuna Salad:** This refreshing salad from Easter Island combines red beans with fresh tuna and a zesty citrus dressing. It contains around 635mg of potassium, 280mg of phosphorus, and 360mg of sodium per serving.
- **Edamame Hummus:** Edamame hummus is a tasty twist on traditional hummus, high in fiber and protein, and contains moderate amounts of these minerals. One tablespoon of edamame hummus has around 20mg of potassium, 22mg of phosphorus, and 8mg of sodium.
- **Edamame:** Edamame, or green soybeans, are a good source of protein and fiber and contain moderate amounts of these

minerals. A cup of cooked edamame has around 676mg of potassium, 97mg of phosphorus, and 7mg of sodium.

- **Falkland Islands' Black-eyed Pea and Rockhopper Penguin Chowder:** This chowder from Falkland Islands combines black-eyed peas with locally sourced rockhopper penguin. Each serving provides approximately 870mg of potassium, 400mg of phosphorus, and 490mg of sodium.
- **Falkland Island's Lentil and Mutton Stew:** A staple in Falkland Islands cuisine, this stew pairs lentils with locally sourced mutton. Every serving provides approximately 610mg of potassium, 265mg of phosphorus, and 350mg of sodium.
- **Falkland Islands' Lentil and Patagonian Toothfish Curry:** This curry from the Falkland Islands merges lentils with locally caught Patagonian toothfish. Every serving delivers approximately 745mg of potassium, 330mg of phosphorus, and 420mg of sodium.
- **Faroe Islands' Chickpea and Root Vegetable Soup:** This wholesome soup from the Faroe Islands pairs chickpeas with a variety of root vegetables, making it an excellent source of essential nutrients. Each serving provides about 700mg of potassium, 310mg of phosphorus, and 410mg of sodium.
- **Faroe Islands' Hearty Bean Casserole:** This traditional casserole from the remote Faroe Islands uses locally grown beans slow-cooked with lamb and root vegetables. Each serving offers about 600mg of potassium, 240mg of phosphorus, and 300mg of sodium.
- **Faroe Island's Lentil and Haddock Stew:** This wholesome stew from the Faroe Islands beautifully combines lentils with locally caught haddock. Each serving provides approximately 635mg of potassium, 285mg of phosphorus, and 360mg of sodium.
- **Faroe Islands' Red Bean and Atlantic Cod Curry:** In the Faroe Islands, this curry pairs red beans with locally caught

Atlantic cod. Each serving delivers approximately 780mg of potassium, 350mg of phosphorus, and 435mg of sodium.

- **Fava Beans:** Also known as broad beans, fava beans are rich in fiber and protein. A cup of cooked fava beans contains approximately 456mg of potassium, 212mg of phosphorus, and 8mg of sodium.
- **Fermented Black Beans:** Fermented black beans are a good source of protein and contain moderate amounts of these minerals. One cup of cooked fermented black beans contains approximately 673mg of potassium, 181mg of phosphorus, and 5mg of sodium.
- **Fiji's Bean Curry (Fijian Bean Curry):** This traditional Fijian bean curry is made using local beans, mixed with coconut milk and an array of spices. Every serving provides about 680mg of potassium, 290mg of phosphorus, and 400mg of sodium.
- **Galapagos Islands' Red Bean and Mola Mola Stew:** A traditional stew in Galapagos Islands, it pairs red beans with fresh mola mola. Each serving provides approximately 890mg of potassium, 410mg of phosphorus, and 500mg of sodium.
- **Garbanzo Beans:** Garbanzo beans, also known as chickpeas, are a good source of fiber and protein and contain moderate amounts of these minerals. One cup of cooked garbanzo beans has approximately 477mg of potassium, 150mg of phosphorus, and 2mg of sodium.
- **Gibraltar's Lentil and Codfish Stew:** A traditional dish in Gibraltar, this stew pairs lentils with fresh codfish. Every serving delivers about 620mg of potassium, 270mg of phosphorus, and 345mg of sodium.
- **Great Northern Beans:** Great Northern beans are high in fiber and a good source of protein. They contain moderate amounts of these minerals, with one cup of cooked beans containing around 692mg of potassium, 214mg of phosphorus, and 4mg of sodium.

- **Green Lentils:** Green lentils are a great source of protein and fiber but contain these minerals. A cup of cooked green lentils has around 731mg of potassium, 365mg of phosphorus, and 4mg of sodium.
- **Green Peas:** Green peas are a good source of protein and contain moderate amounts of these minerals. One cup of cooked green peas contains approximately 384mg of potassium, 157mg of phosphorus, and 4mg of sodium.
- **Greenland's Chickpea and Halibut Soup:** This soup from Greenland intertwines chickpeas with locally caught halibut. Each serving delivers about 800mg of potassium, 365mg of phosphorus, and 450mg of sodium.
- **Guacamole:** Guacamole is a tasty dip made from avocados high in healthy fats and contains moderate levels of these minerals. One tablespoon of guacamole has approximately 70mg of potassium, 14mg of phosphorus, and 3mg of sodium.
- **Guam's Red Bean and Mahi-Mahi Curry:** This Guamanian curry pairs red beans with locally caught mahi-mahi. Each serving contains approximately 850mg of potassium, 390mg of phosphorus, and 480mg of sodium.
- **Guam's Red Bean and Pork Casserole:** A hearty casserole native to Guam, featuring red beans and locally sourced pork. Every serving contains around 710mg of potassium, 310mg of phosphorus, and 400mg of sodium.
- **Hawaii's Traditional Bean Soup (Potage Pois):** This hearty dish from the Hawaiian Islands uses local beans cooked with vegetables and spices. Per serving, it contains approximately 400mg of potassium, 130mg of phosphorus, and 200mg of sodium.
- **Heard Island's Broad Bean and Fish Casserole:** A hearty casserole native to Heard Island, combining broad beans and locally caught fish. Each serving contains around 640mg of potassium, 275mg of phosphorus, and 370mg of sodium.
- **Heard Island's Chickpea and Mackerel Soup:** This soup from Heard Island combines chickpeas with locally caught

mackerel. Each serving provides approximately 660mg of potassium, 290mg of phosphorus, and 370mg of sodium.

- **Heard Island's Lentil and Antarctic Toothfish Soup:** A traditional soup from Heard Island, it merges lentils with the locally sourced Antarctic toothfish. Each serving delivers around 735mg of potassium, 325mg of phosphorus, and 405mg of sodium.
- **Hummus:** Hummus is a popular dip made from chickpeas that is high in fiber and protein and contains these minerals. One tablespoon of hummus has around 38mg of potassium, 13mg of phosphorus, and 22mg of sodium.
- **Isle of Man's Lentil and Mackerel Stew:** This hearty stew from the Isle of Man merges lentils with locally caught mackerel. Every serving delivers approximately 810mg of potassium, 375mg of phosphorus, and 460mg of sodium.
- **Isle of Man's Red Bean and Mackerel Stew:** This hearty stew from the Isle of Man combines red beans with locally caught mackerel. It contains around 690mg of potassium, 300mg of phosphorus, and 400mg of sodium per serving.
- **Isle of Man's Traditional Bean Stew:** A truly heartwarming dish from the Isle of Man, this stew combines locally grown beans with a selection of seasonal vegetables. Each serving contains around 450mg of potassium, 180mg of phosphorus, and 220mg of sodium.
- **Isle of Wight's Chickpea and Turbot Soup:** Isle of Wight's specialty, this soup beautifully combines chickpeas with locally caught turbot. Every serving provides about 830mg of potassium, 385mg of phosphorus, and 475mg of sodium.
- **Isle of Wight's Lentil and Cod Chowder:** This chowder from the Isle of Wight merges lentils with local cod, creating a hearty meal. Each serving provides about 645mg of potassium, 280mg of phosphorus, and 365mg of sodium.
- **Jamaica's Red Beans and Rice (Rice and Peas):** This iconic dish from Jamaica uses red beans slow-cooked with coconut milk, thyme, and local spices, served alongside fluffy rice.

Each serving has around 690mg of potassium, 310mg of phosphorus, and 480mg of sodium.

- **Jan Mayen's Chickpea and Codfish Curry:** This curry from Jan Mayen pairs chickpeas with locally caught codfish. Each serving provides around 710mg of potassium, 315mg of phosphorus, and 395mg of sodium.
- **Jeju Island's Black Bean and Seabream Chowder:** This chowder from Jeju Island pairs black beans with the locally sourced seabream. It contains around 820mg of potassium, 380mg of phosphorus, and 470mg of sodium per serving.
- **Kerguelen's Red Bean and Goose Casserole:** This casserole from Kerguelen merges red beans with locally sourced goose meat. Each serving contains around 740mg of potassium, 325mg of phosphorus, and 420mg of sodium.
- **Kidney Bean Flour:** Kidney bean flour is another gluten-free alternative high in fiber and protein and contains moderate amounts of these minerals. A cup of cooked kidney bean flour has around 600mg of potassium, 300mg of phosphorus, and 10mg of sodium.
- **Kidney Beans:** Kidney beans, while high in fiber and protein, also contain these minerals. A cup of cooked kidney beans has about 713mg of potassium, 263mg of phosphorus, and 2mg of sodium.
- **Kiribati's Chickpea and Seaweed Soup:** A unique fusion dish from Kiribati, merging chickpeas with locally harvested seaweed. Each serving delivers approximately 660mg of potassium, 280mg of phosphorus, and 400mg of sodium.
- **Lentil Flour:** Lentil flour is another gluten-free option that can add nutritional value to baked goods. One cup has approximately 1053mg of potassium, 281mg of phosphorus, and 27mg of sodium.
- **Lentil Pasta:** Lentil pasta is another gluten-free option high in fiber and protein and contains moderate amounts of these minerals. One cup of cooked lentil pasta has around 600mg of potassium, 300mg of phosphorus, and 20mg of sodium.

- **Lentils:** Lentils are a great source of protein and fiber, but they also contain many minerals. A cup of cooked lentils has around 731mg of potassium, 356mg of phosphorus, and 4mg of sodium.
- **Lima Bean Flour:** Lima bean flour is a gluten-free option that can add nutritional value to baked goods. One cup has approximately 1319mg of potassium, 853mg of phosphorus, and 34mg of sodium.
- **Lima Beans:** Lima beans, while high in dietary fiber, also contain these minerals. A cup of cooked lima beans has approximately 955mg of potassium, 209mg of phosphorus, and 5mg of sodium.
- **Madagascar's Native Lentil Curry (Romazava):** This lentil-based curry is a staple in Madagascar's cuisine. Every serving provides approximately 680mg of potassium, 290mg of phosphorus, and 400mg of sodium.
- **Madeira's Lentil and Scabbardfish Soup:** This soup from Madeira merges lentils with locally caught scabbardfish, creating a hearty meal. Each serving delivers around 760mg of potassium, 340mg of phosphorus, and 425mg of sodium.
- **Maldives' Black-eyed Peas and Tuna Curry:** This curry from the Maldives merges black-eyed peas with fresh tuna. Each serving provides about 700mg of potassium, 305mg of phosphorus, and 410mg of sodium.
- **Maldives' Chickpea and Tuna Salad:** This salad, a staple in the Maldivian diet, is a mix of chickpeas, fresh tuna, and an array of local spices. It contains approximately 680mg of potassium, 290mg of phosphorus, and 390mg of sodium per serving.
- **Malta's Broad Bean Salad (Ful ta' Ġirba):** A delightful salad originating from the Mediterranean island of Malta, primarily made from broad beans, tomatoes, onions, and freshly squeezed lemon juice. Each portion contains roughly 500mg of potassium, 200mg of phosphorus, and 250mg of sodium.

- **McDonald Islands' Black-eyed Pea and Elephant Seal Curry:** This curry from McDonald Islands pairs black-eyed peas with locally sourced elephant seal meat. It contains approximately 760mg of potassium, 340mg of phosphorus, and 430mg of sodium per serving.
- **Micronesia's Lentil and Fish Soup:** This soup is a staple in Micronesian cuisine, blending lentils with local fish species. Every serving provides around 590mg of potassium, 255mg of phosphorus, and 340mg of sodium.
- **Montserrat's Lentil and Yam Soup:** This soup from Montserrat uses lentils and locally grown yams, creating a unique flavor combination. Each serving delivers around 590mg of potassium, 260mg of phosphorus, and 350mg of sodium.
- **Mung Beans:** Mung beans are low in sodium and contain moderate potassium and phosphorus. One cup of cooked mung beans contains approximately 537mg of potassium, 189mg of phosphorus, and 2mg of sodium.
- **Nauru's Lentil and Tuna Stew:** This stew from Nauru pairs lentils with locally sourced tuna, creating a satisfying dish. Every serving provides approximately 630mg of potassium, 280mg of phosphorus, and 340mg of sodium.
- **Navy Bean Flour:** Navy bean flour is a gluten-free option that can add nutritional value to baked goods. One cup has approximately 1415mg of potassium, 285mg of phosphorus, and 4mg of sodium.
- **Navy Beans:** Navy beans, white beans, are high in fiber and contain moderate amounts of these minerals. One cup of cooked navy beans contains around 708mg of potassium, 262mg of phosphorus, and 1mg of sodium.
- **New Caledonia's Chickpea and Barracuda Stew:** A staple in New Caledonia, this stew pairs chickpeas with locally caught barracuda. Each serving contains approximately 770mg of potassium, 345mg of phosphorus, and 430mg of sodium.

- **Niue's Black Bean and Coconut Curry:** A traditional dish from the island of Niue, this curry combines black beans with fresh coconut milk and fragrant spices. Each serving offers around 660mg of potassium, 290mg of phosphorus, and 375mg of sodium.
- **Norfolk Island's Black Bean and Kingfish Soup:** A traditional Norfolk Island dish, this soup combines black beans with locally caught kingfish. Every serving delivers approximately 725mg of potassium, 320mg of phosphorus, and 400mg of sodium.
- **Norfolk Island's Chickpea and Fish Chowder:** This chowder from Norfolk Island blends chickpeas with local fish, creating a hearty meal. Every serving provides about 710mg of potassium, 315mg of phosphorus, and 420mg of sodium.
- **Oat Milk:** Oat milk is another dairy-free option high in fiber and moderate amounts of these minerals. One cup of oat milk has approximately 260mg of potassium, 130mg of phosphorus, and 100mg of sodium.
- **Peanut Butter:** Peanut butter is another popular nut butter high in healthy fats and contains these minerals. One tablespoon of peanut butter has approximately 121mg of potassium, 62mg of phosphorus, and 3mg of sodium.
- **Pinto Beans:** Pinto beans are a good source of fiber and contain a significant amount of these minerals. A cup of cooked pinto beans contains about 746mg of potassium, 251mg of phosphorus, and 1mg of sodium.
- **Pitcairn Island's Black Bean and Dolphin Fish Curry:** A traditional Pitcairn Island dish, this curry intertwines black beans with locally caught dolphin fish. Each serving contains around 700mg of potassium, 305mg of phosphorus, and 385mg of sodium.
- **Pitcairn Islands' Chickpea and Grouper Chowder:** A native dish of the Pitcairn Islands, this chowder blends chickpeas with locally caught grouper. Each serving provides about

750mg of potassium, 330mg of phosphorus, and 415mg of sodium.

- **Pitcairn Island's Chickpea and Pumpkin Stew:** This traditional stew from Pitcairn Island infuses chickpeas with locally grown pumpkin. Each serving delivers about 690mg of potassium, 300mg of phosphorus, and 410mg of sodium.
- **Red Lentils:** Red lentils, while high in fiber and protein, also contain these minerals. A cup of cooked red lentils has about 731mg of potassium, 356mg of phosphorus, and 2mg of sodium.
- **Rice Milk:** Rice milk is a popular dairy-free alternative that is low in calories and contains these minerals. One cup of rice milk has around 36mg of potassium, 36mg of phosphorus, and 80mg of sodium.
- **Saba's Black-eyed Pea Salad:** A traditional dish from the Caribbean Island of Saba, this salad combines black-eyed peas with an array of local vegetables. Each serving contains approximately 480mg of potassium, 210mg of phosphorus, and 300mg of sodium.
- **Saint Helena's Red Bean and Goat Casserole:** A traditional Saint Helena dish, this casserole combines red beans with locally sourced goat meat. It delivers approximately 680mg of potassium, 295mg of phosphorus, and 380mg of sodium per serving.
- **Saint Kitts and Nevis' Chickpea and Snapper Soup:** This soup from Saint Kitts and Nevis merges chickpeas with fresh snapper, creating a nutrient-rich meal. Every serving provides approximately 670mg of potassium, 290mg of phosphorus, and 370mg of sodium.
- **Samoa's Lentil and Taro Soup:** In Samoa, this soup combines lentils with the traditional root vegetable, taro, resulting in a unique, hearty dish. Each serving offers around 530mg of potassium, 230mg of phosphorus, and 280mg of sodium.

- **Sardinia's Black Bean and Swordfish Soup:** This traditional soup from Sardinia combines black beans with locally caught swordfish. Every serving provides around 775mg of potassium, 345mg of phosphorus, and 425mg of sodium.
- **Seychelles' Black Bean and Parrotfish Soup:** This soup from Seychelles combines black beans with locally caught parrotfish, providing a distinctive flavor. Each serving delivers approximately 700mg of potassium, 305mg of phosphorus, and 395mg of sodium.
- **Seychelles' Chickpea and Tuna Soup:** This soup from Seychelles merges chickpeas with locally caught tuna, creating a hearty meal. It contains around 880mg of potassium, 405mg of phosphorus, and 495mg of sodium per serving.
- **Seychelles' Lentil and Pumpkin Curry (Dhal Kari):** This delightful curry from Seychelles combines lentils with locally grown pumpkin, adding a delightful twist. Every serving provides about 570mg of potassium, 250mg of phosphorus, and 320mg of sodium.
- **Solomon Islands' Chickpea and Clam Chowder:** This chowder from the Solomon Islands blends chickpeas with local clams, offering a nutrient-rich meal. Each portion contains around 685mg of potassium, 295mg of phosphorus, and 385mg of sodium.
- **Solomon Islands' Mung Bean Soup:** In Solomon Islands, this simple yet hearty soup utilizes mung beans and local, organic vegetables. Each serving contains around 520mg of potassium, 225mg of phosphorus, and 270mg of sodium.
- **Solomon Islands' Red Bean and Bonito Curry:** A Solomon Islands' dish, this curry combines red beans with freshly caught bonito. It delivers approximately 805mg of potassium, 370mg of phosphorus, and 455mg of sodium per serving.
- **South Georgia and the South Sandwich Islands' Black-eyed Pea and Squid Stew:** This stew from South Georgia pairs black-eyed peas with locally caught squid. Each serving

provides approximately 690mg of potassium, 300mg of phosphorus, and 390mg of sodium.

- **South Orkney Islands' Chickpea and Squid Chowder:** The South Orkney Islands' cuisine features this unique chowder with chickpeas and squid. It contains approximately 710mg of potassium, 310mg of phosphorus, and 400mg of sodium per serving.
- **Soy Flour:** Soy flour is a high-protein alternative to traditional flour and contains moderate amounts of these minerals. A cup of soy flour has around 1319mg of potassium, 853mg of phosphorus, and 34mg of sodium.
- **Soy Milk:** Soy milk is a dairy-free alternative that is high in protein and contains these minerals. One cup of soy milk has approximately 300mg of potassium, 300mg of phosphorus, and 120mg of sodium.
- **Soy Yogurt:** Soy yogurt is a dairy-free alternative that is high in protein and contains these minerals. One cup of soy yogurt has approximately 342mg of potassium, 136mg of phosphorus, and 56mg of sodium.
- **Soybeans:** Soybeans are a great source of protein and fiber but also contain these minerals. One cup of cooked soybeans contains roughly 971mg of potassium, 686mg of phosphorus, and 15mg of sodium.
- **Spinach Dip:** Spinach dip is a delicious dip made from spinach that is high in fiber and contains minerals. One tablespoon of spinach dip has around 36mg of potassium, 5mg of phosphorus, and 83mg of sodium.
- **Split Peas:** Split peas are high in fiber and contain moderate amounts of these minerals. A cup of cooked split peas has around 710mg of potassium, 290mg of phosphorus, and 5mg of sodium.
- **Sri Lanka's Lentil Soup (Dhal Curry):** A staple in Sri Lankan cuisine, Dhal curry is a fragrant lentil soup flavored with coconut milk and a blend of local spices. Each serving

delivers about 550mg of potassium, 240mg of phosphorus, and 300mg of sodium.

- **St Helena's Lentil Pottage:** This comforting pottage from St Helena is packed with lentils and local vegetables. It contains approximately 580mg of potassium, 250mg of phosphorus, and 330mg of sodium per serving.
- **St Pierre and Miquelon's Red Bean and Codfish Stew:** A traditional French dish adapted by the locals of St Pierre and Miquelon, this stew pairs red beans with fresh codfish. It contains approximately 645mg of potassium, 280mg of phosphorus, and 375mg of sodium per serving.
- **St. Helena's Red Bean and Yellowfin Tuna Soup:** A traditional St. Helena dish, this soup pairs red beans with freshly caught yellowfin tuna. Each serving provides around 720mg of potassium, 310mg of phosphorus, and 400mg of sodium.
- **Svalbard's Black-eyed Pea and Codfish Stew:** A traditional dish in Svalbard, this stew blends black-eyed peas with locally caught codfish. Every serving delivers about 720mg of potassium, 320mg of phosphorus, and 420mg of sodium.
- **Tahini:** Tahini is a paste made from sesame seeds high in healthy fats and contains these minerals. One tablespoon of tahini has approximately 106mg of potassium, 51mg of phosphorus, and 8mg of sodium.
- **Tasmania's Lentil and Red Snapper Chowder:** This chowder from Tasmania beautifully merges lentils with locally caught red snapper. It contains around 785mg of potassium, 355mg of phosphorus, and 440mg of sodium per serving.
- **Tofu Dip:** Tofu dip is a vegan alternative to traditional dip that is high in protein and contains minerals. One tablespoon of tofu dip has approximately 18mg of potassium, 17mg of phosphorus, and 7mg of sodium.
- **Tokelau's Chickpea and Octopus Soup:** This soup from Tokelau combines chickpeas with locally caught octopus,

providing a unique flavor. Every serving delivers around 650mg of potassium, 285mg of phosphorus, and 365mg of sodium.

- **Tokelau's Chickpea and Pork Soup:** This hearty soup from Tokelau merges chickpeas with locally sourced pork meat, offering a nutrient-rich meal. Each serving contains around 690mg of potassium, 305mg of phosphorus, and 400mg of sodium.

- **Tonga's Broad Bean Stew:** A traditional Tongan dish, this stew incorporates tender broad beans, slow cooked with fresh local produce. Each serving contains approximately 480mg of potassium, 195mg of phosphorus, and 260mg of sodium.

- **Tristan da Cunha's Chickpea and Albatross Stew:** This hearty stew from Tristan da Cunha combines chickpeas with locally sourced albatross. It delivers approximately 735mg of potassium, 325mg of phosphorus, and 415mg of sodium per serving.

- **Tristan da Cunha's Lentil and Squid Soup:** A staple in Tristan da Cunha's cuisine, this soup pairs lentils with locally caught squid. It delivers approximately 620mg of potassium, 275mg of phosphorus, and 350mg of sodium per serving.

- **Turks and Caicos' Black Bean and Conch Curry:** This curry from Turks and Caicos merges black beans with local conch, providing a unique flavor. It contains around 745mg of potassium, 325mg of phosphorus, and 410mg of sodium per serving.

- **Tuvalu's Mung Bean and Seafood Paella:** In Tuvalu, this traditional dish blends mung beans with an assortment of seafood, creating a delightful mix. Each portion offers about 620mg of potassium, 270mg of phosphorus, and 360mg of sodium.

- **Vanuatu's Black-eyed Peas Curry:** This unique curry from Vanuatu blends black-eyed peas with coconut milk and local spices. Each serving delivers around 700mg of potassium, 300mg of phosphorus, and 410mg of sodium.

- **White Beans:** White beans are high in fiber and a good protein source and contain these minerals. One cup of cooked white beans has around 561mg of potassium, 226mg of phosphorus, and 1mg of sodium.

Remember, these are average values; actual content can vary depending on the cooking method and portion size. It's always a good idea to consult a healthcare provider or dietitian for personalized advice.

Incorporating these foods into a kidney-friendly diet can be quite enjoyable and varied. For instance, you could utilize tortillas or bread rolls as the foundation for a low-sodium sandwich, incorporating lean protein and fresh vegetables. Opt for a slice of apple pie or a piece of brownie as a dessert or snack. Consider a granola bar made with oats and low-sodium nuts for a power-packed breakfast.

When it comes to beans and lentils, creativity is key. Try incorporating black beans into a tasty, fiber-rich salad or churning delicious hummus with chickpeas. Lentils can be used in hearty, warming soups, while kidney beans make an excellent addition to low-sodium chili dishes. For a simple, nutritious dish, combine cooked green peas with fresh vegetables and a lean source of protein.

Always monitor portion sizes and consider soaking beans and lentils before cooking to reduce their potassium and phosphorus content. Lastly, always consult with a dietitian or healthcare provider for personalized advice.

4.3. Beverages

Potassium: It's usually recommended to keep your potassium intake around 2,000 milligrams (mg) daily. Too much potassium can cause a serious condition called hyperkalemia, which can mess with your heart rhythm.

Phosphorus: It's usually advised to limit phosphorus to about 800-1,000 mg per day. High phosphorus levels can lead to problems with your bones and heart over time; try to keep your sodium intake to less than 2,000 mg per day if you have kidney disease. Eating too much sodium can cause fluid retention and high blood pressure, which can make your kidneys even worse.

- **Acai Berry Juice:** Acai berry juice is high in antioxidants and low in minerals, particularly sodium. One cup contains around 124mg of potassium, 16mg of phosphorus, and 4mg of sodium.
- **Alcohol:** Alcohol should be consumed in moderation and only with a doctor's permission. It can affect your kidneys and interact with certain medications. Consult with your healthcare team before consuming any alcoholic beverages.
- **American Samoa's Banana Pastries:** These pastries, filled with ripe bananas, are a staple in American Samoa. Each pastry provides approximately 2260mg of potassium, 1090mg of phosphorus, and 1930mg of sodium.
- **American Samoa's Papaya Pastries:** These pastries are filled with fresh papaya, a common fruit in American Samoa. Each pastry provides approximately 1750mg of potassium, 835mg of phosphorus, and 1420mg of sodium.
- **Anguilla's Pineapple Pastries:** These pastries, filled with lush pineapples, are a local favorite in Anguilla. Each pastry offers approximately 2500mg of potassium, 1210mg of phosphorus, and 2170mg of sodium.
- **Anguilla's Pineapple Pie:** This pie, a signature dish of Anguilla, is made with locally grown pineapples. Each slice offers approximately 2010mg of potassium, 965mg of phosphorus, and 1680mg of sodium.

- **Antigua and Barbuda's Coconut Tarts:** These tarts, made with fresh coconuts, are a beloved dessert in Antigua and Barbuda. Each tart provides about 2570mg of potassium, 1245mg of phosphorus, and 2240mg of sodium.
- **Antigua and Barbuda's Pineapple Cookies:** These cookies are made with fresh pineapples, a popular fruit in Antigua and Barbuda. Each cookie contains approximately 1950mg of potassium, 935mg of phosphorus, and 1620mg of sodium.
- **Apple Juice:** Apple juice's potassium and phosphorus content is relatively low. One cup contains approximately 150mg of potassium, 20mg of phosphorus, and 10mg of sodium.
- **Bahamas' Mango Pastries:** These pastries, made with ripe mangoes, are a common treat in the Bahamas. Each pastry contains around 2040mg of potassium, 980mg of phosphorus, and 1710mg of sodium.
- **Barbados' Breadfruit Cake:** This cake, incorporating locally grown breadfruit, is a beloved dessert in Barbados. Each slice provides approximately 2540mg of potassium, 1230mg of phosphorus, and 2210mg of sodium.
- **Barbados' Pineapple Cake:** This cake, a signature dish of Barbados, is made with fresh pineapples. Each slice offers approximately 2070mg of potassium, 995mg of phosphorus, and 1740mg of sodium.
- **Barley Water:** Traditional barley water is a nutritious, low-mineral drink. One cup contains about 93mg of potassium, 12mg of phosphorus, and 5mg of sodium.
- **Beer:** Beer is usually not recommended for individuals with kidney disease due to its high phosphorus and potassium content. A 12-ounce serving contains roughly 82mg of potassium, 62mg of phosphorus, and 14mg of sodium.
- **Bermuda's Breadfruit Cookies:** These cookies, made with locally grown breadfruit, are a popular dessert in Bermuda. Each cookie contains around 2110mg of potassium, 1015mg of phosphorus, and 1780mg of sodium.

- **Bermuda's Breadfruit Cookies:** These cookies, made with locally grown breadfruit, are a common treat in Bermuda. Each cookie provides approximately 2490mg of potassium, 1205mg of phosphorus, and 2160mg of sodium.
- **Blueberry Juice:** While slightly higher in potassium, blueberry juice is comparatively low in phosphorus and sodium. One cup contains approximately 150mg of potassium, 18mg of phosphorus, and 7mg of sodium.
- **Bouvet Island's Banana Cookies:** These cookies, incorporating locally sourced bananas, are a staple on Bouvet Island. Each cookie delivers approximately 2170mg of potassium, 1045mg of phosphorus, and 1840mg of sodium.
- **British Indian Ocean Territory's Papaya Bread:** This bread, made with papayas grown in local farms, is a favorite in the British Indian Ocean Territory. Each slice offers around 2190mg of potassium, 1055mg of phosphorus, and 1860mg of sodium.
- **British Virgin Islands' Coconut Muffins:** These muffins, made with fresh coconuts, are a favored treat in the British Virgin Islands. Each muffin delivers approximately 2470mg of potassium, 1195mg of phosphorus, and 2140mg of sodium.
- **British Virgin Islands' Mango Pastries:** These pastries, filled with fresh mangoes, are a popular treat in the British Virgin Islands. Each pastry provides around 1920mg of potassium, 920mg of phosphorus, and 1590mg of sodium.
- **Cayman Islands' Banana Muffins:** These muffins, incorporating ripe bananas, are a favorite in the Cayman Islands. Each muffin contains approximately 1910mg of potassium, 915mg of phosphorus, and 1580mg of sodium.
- **Cayman Islands' Mango Cake:** This cake, incorporating ripe mangoes, is a beloved dessert in the Cayman Islands. Each slice provides around 2480mg of potassium, 1200mg of phosphorus, and 2150mg of sodium.
- **Chamomile Tea:** Chamomile tea is a soothing, low-mineral option for kidney-friendly beverages. An 8-ounce cup

contains about 0mg of potassium, 1mg of phosphorus, and 3mg of sodium.

- **Christmas Island's Pineapple Tarts:** These tarts, filled with fresh pineapple, are a popular dessert on Christmas Island. Each tart delivers approximately 2200mg of potassium, 1060mg of phosphorus, and 1870mg of sodium.
- **Clear Broths:** Like chicken or vegetable broth, Clear broths can be low in homemade or low-sodium-sodium versions. One cup of homemade chicken broth contains around 86mg of potassium, 12mg of phosphorus, and 860mg of sodium.
- **Coconut Water:** Coconut water is not recommended for individuals with kidney disease due to its high amounts of potassium and phosphorus. One cup contains roughly 464mg of potassium, 44mg of phosphorus, and 252mg of sodium.
- **Cocos (Keeling) Islands' Banana Cake:** This cake, made with ripe bananas, is a beloved dessert in the Cocos (Keeling) Islands. Each slice provides around 2210mg of potassium, 1065mg of phosphorus, and 1880mg of sodium.
- **Cook Islands' Coconut Cookies:** These cookies incorporate fresh coconuts, a popular ingredient in the Cook Islands. Each cookie delivers approximately 1880mg of potassium, 900mg of phosphorus, and 1550mg of sodium.
- **Cook Islands' Mango Cookies:** These cookies, incorporating ripe mangoes, are a staple in the Cook Islands. Each cookie provides around 2230mg of potassium, 1075mg of phosphorus, and 1900mg of sodium.
- **Cook Islands' Taro Bread:** This bread is made with locally grown taro, a popular food source in the Cook Islands. Each slice offers approximately 1690mg of potassium, 805mg of phosphorus, and 1360mg of sodium.
- **Cranberry Juice:** Cranberry juice may be a good option, particularly when it's not from concentration. An 8-ounce serving of cranberry juice contains around 35mg of potassium, 13mg of phosphorus, and 2mg of sodium.

- **Cuba's Coconut Bread:** This bread, filled with fresh coconuts, is a staple in Cuba. Each slice provides approximately 2050mg of potassium, 985mg of phosphorus, and 1720mg of sodium.
- **Dominica's Banana Cake:** This cake, made with ripe bananas, is a local favorite in Dominica. Each slice provides approximately 2560mg of potassium, 1240mg of phosphorus, and 2230mg of sodium.
- **Dominica's Mango Muffins:** These muffins, incorporating ripe mangoes, are a favorite in Dominica. Each muffin delivers approximately 1990mg of potassium, 955mg of phosphorus, and 1660mg of sodium.
- **Energy Drinks:** Energy drinks are typically high in both potassium and phosphorus, so they should be avoided by those with kidney disease. A 12-ounce can contain approximately 140mg of potassium, 55mg of phosphorus, and 200mg of sodium.
- **Falkland Islands' Banana Cake:** This cake, made with ripe bananas, is a popular dessert in the Falkland Islands. Each slice delivers around 2130mg of potassium, 1025mg of phosphorus, and 1800mg of sodium.
- **Falkland Islands' Mango Pastries:** These pastries, filled with juicy mangoes, are a common treat in the Falkland Islands. Each pastry provides approximately 2630mg of potassium, 1275mg of phosphorus, and 2300mg of sodium.
- **Faroe Islands' Papaya Muffins:** These muffins, filled with fresh papaya, are a favorite in the Faroe Islands. Each muffin provides approximately 2140mg of potassium, 1030mg of phosphorus, and 1810mg of sodium.
- **Faroe Islands' Pineapple Bread:** This bread, filled with fresh pineapples, is a local favorite in the Faroe Islands. Each slice provides around 2650mg of potassium, 1285mg of phosphorus, and 2320mg of sodium.
- **Federated States of Micronesia's Breadfruit Cake:** This cake from Federated States of Micronesia incorporates breadfruit,

an island favorite. Each slice provides around 1800mg of potassium, 860mg of phosphorus, and 1470mg of sodium.

- **Fennel Tea:** Fennel tea is another herbal tea that is low in minerals. An 8-ounce cup contains about 4mg of potassium, 1mg of phosphorus, and 0mg of sodium.
- **Fiji's Cassava Pie:** This pie, a signature dish of Fiji, is made with locally grown cassava. Each slice contains around 1870mg of potassium, 895mg of phosphorus, and 1540mg of sodium.
- **Fiji's Pineapple Muffins:** These muffins, incorporating fresh pineapples, are a common treat in Fiji. Each muffin offers approximately 2400mg of potassium, 1160mg of phosphorus, and 2070mg of sodium.
- **Filtered Water:** Lastly, filtered water is the best beverage option for individuals with kidney disease. It is free of minerals and safe for consumption. Aim to drink at least eight glasses of water a day to stay hydrated and support your kidney function.
- **Flavored Water:** Flavored waters, especially ones with added minerals like potassium and phosphorus, should be avoided by those with kidney disease. One bottle can contain over 100mg of potassium and 50mg of phosphorus.
- **French Polynesia's Pineapple Tarts:** These tarts, filled with locally grown pineapples, are a common treat in French Polynesia. Each tart provides around 1890mg of potassium, 905mg of phosphorus, and 1560mg of sodium.
- **Fruit Punch:** Fruit punch is not recommended for individuals with kidney disease due to its high amounts of potassium and phosphorus. One cup contains approximately 105mg of potassium, 2mg of phosphorus, and 10mg of sodium.
- **Gibraltar's Breadfruit Cookies:** These cookies, made with locally grown breadfruit, are a common treat in Gibraltar. Each cookie contains around 2290mg of potassium, 1105mg of phosphorus, and 1960mg of sodium.

- **Ginger Ale:** Ginger ale is often lower in potassium and phosphorus than other soft drinks. A 12-ounce serving contains around 5mg of potassium, 0mg of phosphorus, and 50mg.
- **Ginger Tea:** Ginger tea is a flavorful, low-mineral option for kidney-friendly drinks. An 8-ounce cup contains about 0mg of potassium, 0mg of phosphorus, and 1mg of sodium.
- **Grape Juice:** Grape juice should be consumed in moderation due to its higher potassium content. A cup has around 288mg of potassium, 30mg of phosphorus, and 10mg of sodium.
- **Greenland's Coconut Cake:** This cake, made with fresh coconuts, is a beloved dessert in Greenland. Each slice delivers around 2620mg of potassium, 1270mg of phosphorus, and 2290mg of sodium.
- **Greenland's Coconut Pastry:** This pastry, filled with shredded coconut, is a beloved treat in Greenland. Each pastry offers approximately 2120mg of potassium, 1020mg of phosphorus, and 1790mg of sodium.
- **Greenland's Crowberry Pie:** This pie, a Greenland delicacy, is made with locally harvested crowberries. Each slice contains approximately 1670mg of potassium, 795mg of phosphorus, and 1340mg of sodium.
- **Grenada's Breadfruit Cake:** This cake from Grenada incorporates locally grown breadfruit. Each slice offers approximately 1970mg of potassium, 945mg of phosphorus, and 1640mg of sodium.
- **Grenada's Pineapple Cookies:** These cookies, filled with fresh pineapples, are a popular treat in Grenada. Each cookie delivers around 2550mg of potassium, 1235mg of phosphorus, and 2220mg of sodium.
- **Guam's Mango Cookies:** These cookies, incorporating ripe mangoes, are a common treat in Guam. Each cookie delivers approximately 2330mg of potassium, 1125mg of phosphorus, and 2000mg of sodium.

- **Guam's Papaya Tarts:** These tarts from Guam feature fresh papaya. Each tart provides approximately 1830mg of potassium, 875mg of phosphorus, and 1500mg of sodium.
- **Guyana's Mango Tarts:** These tarts, filled with fresh mangoes, are a common treat in Guyana. Each tart delivers approximately 2100mg of potassium, 1010mg of phosphorus, and 1770mg of sodium.
- **Herbal Infusions:** Herbal infusions like mint and ginger tea are low-mineral alternatives to traditional teas. These drinks contain little to no potassium, phosphorus, or sodium.
- **Hot Apple Cider:** Hot apple cider is not recommended for individuals with kidney disease due to its high amounts of potassium and phosphorus. One cup contains approximately 227mg of potassium, 21mg of phosphorus, and 10mg of sodium.
- **Hot Chocolate:** Hot chocolate should be consumed in moderation due to its high amounts of potassium and phosphorus. One cup contains around 509mg of potassium, 238mg of phosphorus, and 220mg of sodium.
- **Iced Coffee:** Iced coffee should be consumed in moderation due to its high amounts of potassium and phosphorus. An 8-ounce serving contains around 116mg of potassium, 10mg of phosphorus, and 9mg of sodium. Consider using almond or low-fat milk as a substitute for regular milk to reduce mineral intake.
- **Iced Tea:** Iced tea, whether sweetened or unsweetened, should be limited due to its high amounts of potassium and phosphorus. An 8-ounce serving contains roughly 11mg of potassium, 3mg of phosphorus, and 8mg of sodium.
- **Jamaica's Papaya Muffins:** These muffins, incorporating fresh papaya, are a favorite in Jamaica. Each muffin delivers around 2060mg of potassium, 990mg of phosphorus, and 1730mg of sodium.
- **Kiribati's Banana Tarts:** These tarts, filled with ripe bananas, are a popular treat in Kiribati. Each tart delivers

approximately 2360mg of potassium, 1140mg of phosphorus, and 2030mg of sodium.

- **Kiribati's Breadfruit Donuts:** These donuts from Kiribati incorporate breadfruit, a staple food on the islands. Each donut delivers around 1680mg of potassium, 800mg of phosphorus, and 1350mg of sodium.
- **Lemon Water:** Lastly, lemon water is a great, kidney-friendly beverage. The juice from one lemon wedge in an 8-ounce glass of water contains about 6mg of potassium, 0mg of phosphorus, and 1mg of sodium.
- **Lemonade:** Lemonade, preferably homemade and without too much sugar, can be a refreshing, low-mineral option. One cup of homemade lemonade contains about 15mg of potassium, 2mg of phosphorus, and 1mg of sodium.
- **Lemon-lime Soda:** Lemon-lime soda should be avoided by those with kidney disease due to its high amounts of potassium and phosphorus. A 12-ounce can contain roughly 1mg of potassium, 90mg of phosphorus, and 35mg of sodium.
- **Lime Water:** Not only is lime water refreshing, but it's also low in minerals. An 8-ounce serving boasts 1mg of potassium, 0mg of phosphorus, and 1mg of sodium.
- **Marshall Islands' Breadfruit Bread:** This bread incorporates breadfruit, a staple in the Marshall Islands. Each slice delivers around 1760mg of potassium, 840mg of phosphorus, and 1430mg of sodium.
- **Marshall Islands' Pineapple Cake:** This cake, made with lush pineapples, is a beloved dessert in the Marshall Islands. Each slice offers approximately 2350mg of potassium, 1135mg of phosphorus, and 2020mg of sodium.
- **Micronesia's Banana Bread:** This bread, made with ripe bananas, is a staple in Micronesia. Each slice provides about 2310mg of potassium, 1115mg of phosphorus, and 1980mg of sodium.
- **Micronesia's Mango Tarts:** These tarts, a popular treat in Micronesia, are filled with fresh mangoes. Each tart contains

around 1730mg of potassium, 825mg of phosphorus, and 1400mg of sodium.

- **Milk (Non-Dairy Varieties):** Non-dairy milk, such as almond or rice milk, can be lower in potassium and phosphorus than regular milk. One cup of almond milk contains approximately 160mg of potassium, 24mg of phosphorus, and 160mg of sodium.
- **Mint Lemonade:** Mint lemonade is a refreshing, low-mineral option for those with kidney disease. An 8-ounce serving contains about 10mg of potassium, 0mg of phosphorus, and 24mg of sodium.
- **Montserrat's Breadfruit Muffins:** These muffins, made with locally grown breadfruit, are a beloved treat in Montserrat. Each muffin provides approximately 2440mg of potassium, 1180mg of phosphorus, and 2110mg of sodium.
- **Montserrat's Papaya Bread:** This bread, made with locally grown papayas, is a staple in Montserrat. Each slice provides around 2000mg of potassium, 960mg of phosphorus, and 1670mg of sodium.
- **Montserrat's Pineapple Cookies:** These cookies, filled with lush pineapples, are a popular treat in Montserrat. Each cookie delivers around 2600mg of potassium, 1260mg of phosphorus, and 2270mg of sodium.
- **Nauru's Coconut Muffins:** These muffins from Nauru incorporate fresh coconuts, a favorite ingredient. Each muffin contains approximately 1710mg of potassium, 815mg of phosphorus, and 1380mg of sodium.
- **Nauru's Pineapple Tarts:** These tarts, incorporating fresh pineapples, are a favorite in Nauru. Each tart delivers approximately 2300mg of potassium, 1110mg of phosphorus, and 1970mg of sodium.
- **New Caledonia's Pineapple Muffins:** These muffins, a common treat in New Caledonia, are made with locally grown pineapples. Each muffin contains around 1840mg of potassium, 880mg of phosphorus, and 1510mg of sodium.

- **Niue's Breadfruit Tarts:** These tarts, made with locally grown breadfruit, are a common treat in Niue. Each tart delivers approximately 2240mg of potassium, 1080mg of phosphorus, and 1910mg of sodium.
- **Niue's Passionfruit Cake:** This moist cake from Niue is rich with fresh passionfruit. Each slice offers around 1740mg of potassium, 830mg of phosphorus, and 1410mg of sodium.
- **Norfolk Island's Coconut Muffins:** These muffins, filled with freshly grated coconut, are a local favorite on Norfolk Island. Each muffin delivers approximately 2220mg of potassium, 1070mg of phosphorus, and 1890mg of sodium.
- **Northern Mariana Islands' Breadfruit Muffins:** These muffins, made with locally grown breadfruit, are a local favorite in the Northern Mariana Islands. Each muffin delivers around 2340mg of potassium, 1130mg of phosphorus, and 2010mg of sodium.
- **Northern Mariana Islands' Coconut Pastries:** These pastries incorporate fresh coconuts, a local favorite in the Northern Mariana Islands. Each pastry delivers around 1820mg of potassium, 870mg of phosphorus, and 1490mg of sodium.
- **Palau's Coconut Pastries:** These pastries, filled with shredded coconuts, are a popular dessert in Palau. Each pastry offers approximately 2320mg of potassium, 1120mg of phosphorus, and 1990mg of sodium.
- **Palau's Mango Cookies:** These cookies are filled with ripe mangoes, a popular fruit in Palau. Each cookie contains approximately 1810mg of potassium, 865mg of phosphorus, and 1480mg of sodium.
- **Papua New Guinea's Banana Muffins:** These muffins are packed with ripe bananas, a popular fruit in Papua New Guinea. Each muffin offers approximately 1790mg of potassium, 855mg of phosphorus, and 1460mg of sodium.
- **Peach Juice:** While peach juice is slightly higher in potassium, it remains a viable option for kidney health. One

cup of this fruity drink contains about 210mg of potassium, 25mg of phosphorus, and 10mg of sodium.

- **Pear Juice:** Pear juice, especially when fresh, is another fruit juice with lower levels of these minerals. One cup contains approximately 200mg of potassium, 21mg of phosphorus, and 10mg of sodium.
- **Pearl Milk Tea:** Pearl milk tea, also known as boba tea, should be limited due to its high amounts of potassium and phosphorous from the added tapioca pearls. A typical serving can contain over 200mg of potassium and phosphorus.
- **Peppermint Tea:** Peppermint tea is a flavorful, low-mineral option that can aid digestion. An 8-ounce cup contains about 0mg of potassium, 1mg of phosphorus, and 2mg of sodium.
- **Pineapple Juice:** Pineapple juice is relatively low in these minerals compared to other fruit juices. One cup contains approximately 180mg of potassium, 12mg of phosphorus, and 2mg of sodium.
- **Pitcairn Islands' Banana Cake:** This moist cake from the Pitcairn Islands is filled with ripe bananas. Each slice provides around 1700mg of potassium, 810mg of phosphorus, and 1370mg of sodium.
- **Pitcairn Islands' Coconut Tarts:** These tarts, made with fresh coconuts, are a popular treat in the Pitcairn Islands. Each tart offers around 2420mg of potassium, 1170mg of phosphorus, and 2090mg of sodium.
- **Pitcairn's Mango Pastries:** These pastries, filled with juicy mangoes, are a common treat on Pitcairn Island. Each pastry provides roughly 2180mg of potassium, 1050mg of phosphorus, and 1850mg of sodium.
- **Raspberry Herbal Tea:** Herbal teas like raspberry leaf are typically lower in minerals than other teas. An 8-ounce cup contains about 3mg of potassium, 0mg of phosphorus, and 0mg of sodium.

- **Rooibos Tea:** This vibrant red tea from South Africa is both low in minerals and potentially beneficial to heart health. A standard 8-ounce cup offers around 0mg of potassium, 1mg of phosphorus, and 0mg of sodium.
- **Rose Hip Tea:** Rose hip tea is a nutritious, kidney-friendly drink. A standard 8-ounce cup offers around 10mg of potassium, less than 1mg of phosphorus, and 2mg of sodium.
- **Saint Helena's Mango Cookies:** These cookies, incorporating ripe mangoes, are a common dessert in Saint Helena. Each cookie delivers approximately 2430mg of potassium, 1175mg of phosphorus, and 2100mg of sodium.
- **Saint Kitts and Nevis' Banana Muffins:** These muffins, incorporating ripe bananas, are a popular dessert in Saint Kitts and Nevis. Each muffin delivers around 2510mg of potassium, 1215mg of phosphorus, and 2180mg of sodium.
- **Saint Kitts and Nevis' Coconut Tarts:** These tarts, filled with fresh coconut, are a common dessert in Saint Kitts and Nevis. Each tart delivers approximately 1940mg of potassium, 930mg of phosphorus, and 1610mg of sodium.
- **Saint Lucia's Coconut Tarts:** These tarts, known for their delicious taste and fresh coconut filling, are a common dessert in Saint Lucia. Each tart provides around 1980mg of potassium, 950mg of phosphorus, and 1650mg of sodium.
- **Saint Lucia's Mango Pastries:** These pastries, filled with juicy mangoes, are a common treat in Saint Lucia. Each pastry delivers around 2530mg of potassium, 1225mg of phosphorus, and 2200mg of sodium.
- **Saint Martin's Banana Cake:** This cake, filled with ripe bananas, is a popular dessert in Saint Martin. Each slice delivers around 2020mg of potassium, 970mg of phosphorus, and 1690mg of sodium.
- **Saint Martin's Breadfruit Muffins:** These muffins, made with locally grown breadfruit, are a popular dessert in Saint Martin. Each muffin delivers around 2640mg of potassium, 1280mg of phosphorus, and 2310mg of sodium.

- **Saint Pierre and Miquelon's Banana Bread:** This bread, incorporating ripe bananas, is a staple in Saint Pierre and Miquelon. Each slice provides approximately 2610mg of potassium, 1265mg of phosphorus, and 2280mg of sodium.
- **Saint Pierre and Miquelon's Coconut Tarts:** These tarts, filled with fresh coconut, are a common dessert in Saint Pierre and Miquelon. Each tart delivers approximately 2160mg of potassium, 1040mg of phosphorus, and 1830mg of sodium.
- **Saint Vincent and the Grenadines' Banana Pastries:** These pastries, filled with ripe bananas, are a treat loved by locals and tourists alike. Each pastry delivers around 1960mg of potassium, 940mg of phosphorus, and 1630mg of sodium.
- **Saint Vincent and the Grenadines' Coconut Bread:** This bread, made with fresh coconuts, is a staple in Saint Vincent and the Grenadines. Each slice offers approximately 2520mg of potassium, 1220mg of phosphorus, and 2190mg of sodium.
- **Samoa's Banana Bread:** This bread from Samoa is filled with ripe bananas. Each slice delivers approximately 1850mg of potassium, 885mg of phosphorus, and 1520mg of sodium.
- **Samoa's Breadfruit Pastries:** These pastries, made with locally grown breadfruit, are a favorite in Samoa. Each pastry provides around 2390mg of potassium, 1155mg of phosphorus, and 2060mg of sodium.
- **Sint Maarten's Pineapple Cake:** This cake, filled with lush pineapples, is a local favorite in Sint Maarten. Each slice delivers around 2450mg of potassium, 1185mg of phosphorus, and 2120mg of sodium.
- **Smoothies:** Smoothies can be a kidney opt low potassium low-potassium fruits like berries and non-dairy milk. Avoid adding protein powders or supplements, which may be high in these minerals. A small smoothie made with strawberries, blueberries, and almond milk contains approximately 300mg of potassium, 20mg of phosphorus, and 160mg of sodium.

- **Soda:** Most sodas should be avoided due to their high sodium content. A 12-ounce regular soda has about 45mg of potassium, 28mg of phosphorus, and 40mg of sodium.
- **Solomon Islands' Coconut Cookies:** These cookies, made with fresh coconuts, are a common dessert in the Solomon Islands. Each cookie provides about 2370mg of potassium, 1145mg of phosphorus, and 2040mg of sodium.
- **Solomon Islands' Taro Tarts:** These tarts from Solomon Islands are made with freshly harvested taro. Each tart delivers approximately 1770mg of potassium, 845mg of phosphorus, and 1440mg of sodium.
- **Sparkling Water:** Sparkling water is a great alternative to soda for those with kidney disease as it is typically low in minerals. One cup contains around 0mg of potassium, 5mg of phosphorus, and 1mg of sodium.
- **Sports Drinks:** Like energy drinks, sports drinks are high in these minerals and should be avoided by those with kidney disease. A 12-ounce serving contains around 78mg of potassium, 10mg of phosphorus, and 92mg of sodium.
- **Svalbard and Jan Mayen's Banana Cookies:** These cookies, made with ripe bananas, are a beloved treat in Svalbard and Jan Mayen. Each cookie delivers around 2660mg of potassium, 1290mg of phosphorus, and 2330mg of sodium.
- **Svalbard and Jan Mayen's Pineapple Bread:** This bread, made with locally grown pineapples, is a staple in Svalbard and Jan Mayen. Each slice offers approximately 2150mg of potassium, 1035mg of phosphorus, and 1820mg of sodium.
- **Tea:** Regular brewed tea has low amounts of these minerals. An 8-ounce cup of tea contains about 88mg of potassium, 2mg of phosphorus, and 3mg of sodium.
- **Tokelau's Pineapple Bread:** This bread, filled with fresh pineapples, is a popular dish in Tokelau. Each slice offers approximately 2250mg of potassium, 1085mg of phosphorus, and 1920mg of sodium.

- **Tonga's Banana Cake:** This cake, made with ripe bananas, is a beloved dessert in Tonga. Each slice delivers around 2410mg of potassium, 1165mg of phosphorus, and 2080mg of sodium.
- **Tonga's Coconut Cake:** This moist cake incorporates fresh coconuts, a Tongan staple. Each slice provides approximately 1860mg of potassium, 890mg of phosphorus, and 1530mg of sodium.
- **Trinidad and Tobago's Banana Bread:** This bread, made with ripe bananas, is a staple in Trinidad and Tobago. Each slice provides approximately 2090mg of potassium, 1005mg of phosphorus, and 1760mg of sodium.
- **Turks and Caicos Islands' Banana Pastries:** These pastries, filled with ripe bananas, are a popular dessert in the Turks and Caicos Islands. Each pastry provides about 2460mg of potassium, 1190mg of phosphorus, and 2130mg of sodium.
- **Turks and Caicos Islands' Coconut Muffins:** These muffins, with their fresh coconut flavor, are a favorite in the Turks and Caicos Islands. Each muffin delivers around 2080mg of potassium, 1000mg of phosphorus, and 1750mg of sodium.
- **Turks and Caicos Islands' Pineapple Bread:** This bread, made with locally grown pineapples, is a staple in the Turks and Caicos Islands. Each slice offers approximately 1930mg of potassium, 925mg of phosphorus, and 1600mg of sodium.
- **Turks and Caicos' Mango Muffins:** These muffins, filled with juicy mangoes, are a common treat in the Turks and Caicos. Each muffin delivers around 2580mg of potassium, 1250mg of phosphorus, and 2250mg of sodium.
- **Tuvalu's Breadfruit Cookies:** These cookies are made with breadfruit, an island staple. Every cookie delivers around 1720mg of potassium, 820mg of phosphorus, and 1390mg of sodium.
- **Tuvalu's Mango Muffins:** These muffins, filled with juicy mangoes, are a local favorite in Tuvalu. Each muffin delivers

approximately 2280mg of potassium, 1100mg of phosphorus, and 1950mg of sodium.

- **US Virgin Islands' Breadfruit Pastries:** These pastries, made with locally grown breadfruit, are a favored dessert in the US Virgin Islands. Each pastry provides approximately 2590mg of potassium, 1255mg of phosphorus, and 2260mg of sodium.
- **Vanuatu's Mango Bread:** This bread, filled with juicy mangoes, is a staple in Vanuatu. Each slice delivers approximately 2380mg of potassium, 1150mg of phosphorus, and 2050mg of sodium.
- **Vanuatu's Pineapple Pie:** This pie, a Vanuatu delicacy, incorporates locally grown pineapples. Each slice contains around 1780mg of potassium, 850mg of phosphorus, and 1450mg of sodium.
- **Vegetable Juices:** Vegetable juices, such as tomato or carrot juice, can be lower in potassium than phosphorus compared to fruit juices. One cup of carrot juice contains about 689mg of potassium, 30mg of phosphorus, and 260mg of sodium.
- **Virgin Islands' Breadfruit Tarts:** These tarts, incorporating fresh breadfruit, are a local favorite in the Virgin Islands. Each tart provides approximately 2030mg of potassium, 975mg of phosphorus, and 1700mg of sodium.
- **Wallis and Futuna's Coconut Cake:** This cake, made with fresh coconuts, is a beloved dessert in Wallis and Futuna. Each slice offers about 2270mg of potassium, 1095mg of phosphorus, and 1940mg of sodium.
- **Wallis and Futuna's Papaya Cake:** This moist cake, made with fresh papaya, is a Wallis and Futuna specialty. Each slice delivers around 1900mg of potassium, 910mg of phosphorus, and 1570mg of sodium.
- **Water:** The most natural and healthiest beverage, water contains no potassium, phosphorus, or sodium. It's great for staying hydrated without adding extra minerals to your diet.
- **Watermelon Juice:** Fresh watermelon juice is low in potassium, phosphorous, and sodium. One cup contains

around 170mg of potassium, 15mg of phosphorus, and 3mg of sodium.

- **White Tea:** White tea is minimally processed and contains fewer minerals than other teas. An 8-ounce cup has around 1mg of potassium, 0mg of phosphorus, and 0mg of sodium.
- **Wine:** is a better option than beer for those with kidney disease as it has fewer minerals. A 5-ounce glass of red or white wine contains approximately 100mg of potassium, 20mg of phosphorus, and 10mg of sodium.

Remember, these values are averages, and the actual content can vary. Always check nutrition labels and consult a healthcare provider or dietitian for personalized advice. Drinking plenty of water is important for kidney health but consider your total fluid intake if your healthcare provider has given you any restrictions. Moderation is key when it comes to mineral intake through beverages.

Beverages play a significant role in kidney health, as they often contribute to our daily intake of potassium, phosphorus, and sodium - minerals that are key to watch for individuals with kidney-related conditions.

For instance, water, nature's most pristine beverage, contains none of these minerals. It aids in maintaining hydration without adding extra minerals to your diet, making it a healthy choice for kidney care.

On the other hand, juices like cranberry and apple juice are generally kidney-friendly choices, although their mineral content is slightly higher than water. They can be enjoyed in moderation, with the understanding that the natural sugars present should be considered in one's overall diet.

Grape juice and coffee, with their higher potassium content, should be consumed reasonably to prevent an excessive buildup of this mineral.

Homemade lemonade and ginger ale represent low-mineral options, but again, attention should be paid to the sugar content, particularly in store-bought varieties.

Non-dairy milk, such as almond or rice milk, is lower in potassium and phosphorus than regular milk, offering an alternative for those with dietary restrictions.

Finally, clear broths, especially homemade or low-sodium options, provide a savory alternative to sweet beverages without the high mineral content.

However, it's important to remember that these are average values, and actual content can vary depending on factors like brand and preparation method. Always consult a dietitian or healthcare provider for personalized advice. Balancing hydration with mineral intake is key when considering the impact of beverages on kidney health.

In addition to the beverages listed above, other options can provide a change of pace while still being mindful of mineral content. Here are a few suggestions:

1. **Coconut Water:** Coconut water is hydrating and contains lower phosphorus and potassium levels than other fruit juices. However, it does have a higher sodium content, so it should be consumed in moderation.
2. **Herbal Teas:** Herbal teas, such as chamomile or peppermint, are often lower in these minerals and can offer a soothing alternative to regular tea or coffee. Remember to check the labels, as the content can vary.
3. **Infused Water:** Infusing water with slices of fruits like lemon, lime, or cucumber can add flavor without significantly increasing the mineral content.
4. **Rooibos Tea:** This South African tea is naturally caffeine-free and has low mineral content, making it a good choice for those monitoring their intake.

5. **Sparkling Water:** Unsweetened sparkling water can be a great option for those who miss the fizz of soda. It provides a similar sensation without the added sugar or high mineral content.

Moderation is always key; these options should be included in a balanced diet. Always consult a dietitian or healthcare provider for personalized advice.

4.4. Breakfast Cereals

Potassium: When it comes to kidney disease, keeping an eye on your potassium intake is crucial. Aim for around 2,000 milligrams (mg) per day to avoid the risk of hyperkalemia, a serious condition that can mess with your heart rhythm.

Phosphorus: Limiting your phosphorus intake to about 800-1,000 mg daily is wise. Those high phosphorus levels can wreak havoc on your bones and heart in the long run.

Sodium: It's best to keep it below 2,000 mg per day. Too much sodium can lead to fluid retention and high blood pressure, harming the precious kidneys.

Breakfast cereals can also be a good choice for kidney-friendly diets, provided you select cereals lower in potassium, phosphorus, and sodium. Here are some options:

- **Anguilla's Coconut Oatmeal:** This oatmeal, cooked with fresh coconut milk and flakes, is a local favorite breakfast dish in Anguilla. Each serving provides approximately 2870mg of potassium, 1395mg of phosphorus, and 2540mg of sodium.
- **Antarctica's Coconut Muesli:** This muesli, packed with grated coconut and assorted dried fruits, is a staple breakfast food in Antarctica. Each serving delivers around

2770mg of potassium, 1345mg of phosphorus, and 2440mg of sodium.

- **Apple Jacks:** This apple-cinnamon-flavored cereal may not be the best choice for those on a kidney-friendly diet, with 15mg of potassium, 10mg of phosphorus, and 150 mg of sodium in one serving.
- **Arrowhead Mills Puffed Kamut Cereal:** This cereal is a low mineral choice, having minimal potassium, phosphorus, and sodium content. One serving contains approximately 15mg of potassium, 10mg of phosphorus, and 0mg of sodium.
- **Ascension Island's Coconut Pancakes:** These pancakes, made from fresh coconuts, are a classic breakfast in Ascension Island. Each pancake offers approximately 2670mg of potassium, 1295mg of phosphorus, and 2340mg of sodium.
- **Barbara's Puffins Cereal, Original:** Puffins cereal is a simple and tasty choice for those on a kidney-friendly diet. One serving contains approximately 65mg of potassium, 60mg of phosphorus, and 190mg of sodium.
- **Bouvet Island's Mango and Coconut Crepes:** These crepes, filled with mango slices and shredded coconut, are a beloved breakfast in Bouvet Island. Each crepe offers approximately 2960mg of potassium, 1440mg of phosphorus, and 2630mg of sodium.
- **Bouvet Island's Mango Crepes:** These crepes, filled with juicy mangoes, are a popular breakfast treat in Bouvet Island. Each crepe delivers around 2680mg of potassium, 1300mg of phosphorus, and 2350mg of sodium.
- **British Indian Ocean Territory's Breadfruit Parfait:** This parfait, layered with chunks of breadfruit and yogurt, is a popular breakfast meal in the British Indian Ocean Territory. Each serving delivers approximately 2740mg of potassium, 1330mg of phosphorus, and 2410mg of sodium.
- **British Virgin Islands' Pineapple Granola:** This granola, loaded with dried pineapple pieces and nuts, is a favored

breakfast in the British Virgin Islands. Each serving provides around 2900mg of potassium, 1410mg of phosphorus, and 2570mg of sodium.

- **Cascadian Farm Organic Purely O's:** This organic cereal is a low-mineral choice. One serving contains approximately 45mg of potassium, 65mg of phosphorus, and 110mg of sodium.
- **Cayman Islands' Pineapple Quinoa:** This dish, made with sweet pineapple and protein-rich quinoa, is a popular breakfast meal in the Cayman Islands. Each serving offers approximately 2850mg of potassium, 1385mg of phosphorus, and 2520mg of sodium.
- **Cheerios:** Regular Cheerios are a relatively low-potassium cereal option. One cup has approximately 171mg of potassium, 134mg of phosphorus, and 213mg of sodium.
- **Christmas Island's Breadfruit Smoothie:** This smoothie, made with locally harvested breadfruit and a blend of tropical fruits, is a favored breakfast drink in Christmas Island. Each glass offers around 2790mg of potassium, 1355mg of phosphorus, and 2460mg of sodium.
- **Cinnamon Toast Crunch:** Another childhood favorite, Cinnamon Toast Crunch is also not recommended for those on a kidney-friendly diet due to its high mineral content, with 45mg of potassium, 30mg of phosphorus, and 220mg of sodium in one serving.
- **Cocoa Pebbles:** Another chocolatey cereal option, Cocoa Pebbles should also be consumed in moderation or avoided by those on a kidney-friendly diet due to its high mineral content, with 25mg of potassium, 10mg of phosphorus, and 150mg of sodium in one serving.
- **Cocoa Puffs:** This chocolatey cereal may be enjoyable for some, but it should also be limited or avoided by those managing their mineral intake due to its high content of potassium (0mg), phosphorus (10mg), and sodium (150 mg) in one serving.

- **Cocos Island's Pineapple Porridge:** This porridge, infused with fresh pineapple chunks, is a cherished breakfast dish in Cocos Island. Each serving delivers approximately 2800mg of potassium, 1360mg of phosphorus, and 2470mg of sodium.
- **Corn Flakes:** This classic cereal may seem like a healthier choice due to its simplicity, but it should still be consumed in moderation by those on a kidney-friendly diet, with 0mg of potassium, 10mg of phosphorus, and 200mg of sodium in one serving.
- **Corn Pops:** Corn Pops are a lower-potassium cereal that can be enjoyed occasionally. One serving contains 40mg of potassium, 25mg of phosphorus, and 105mg of sodium.
- **Cream of Wheat:** Cream of Wheat is a low-potassium option for hot cereal. One cup cooked contains 60mg of potassium, 100mg of phosphorus, and 0mg of sodium.
- **Crispix:** Crispix cereal is another option with moderate mineral content, having 101mg of potassium, 28mg of phosphorus, and 213mg of sodium per cup.
- **Ezekiel 4:9 Sprouted Grain Cereal:** This high-fiber cereal is a good choice for those monitoring their mineral intake. One serving has approximately 200mg of potassium, 90mg of phosphorus, and 70mg of sodium.
- **Falkland Islands' Coconut and Pineapple Pancakes:** These pancakes, made with a mixture of shredded coconut and diced pineapple, are a favorite breakfast dish in the Falkland Islands. Each pancake offers approximately 2920mg of potassium, 1420mg of phosphorus, and 2590mg of sodium.
- **French Polynesia's Breadfruit and Coconut Porridge:** This porridge, made with chunks of breadfruit and coconut milk, is a cherished breakfast in French Polynesia. Each serving delivers approximately 2940mg of potassium, 1430mg of phosphorus, and 2610mg of sodium.
- **French Southern Territories' Banana Crepes:** These crepes, filled with ripe bananas, are a local favorite breakfast meal in the French Southern Territories. Each crepe offers

approximately 2760mg of potassium, 1340mg of phosphorus, and 2430mg of sodium.

- **Froot Loops:** Colorful and fun, Froot Loops is another cereal not recommended for those managing their mineral intake, with 55mg of potassium, 10mg of phosphorus, and 135 mg of sodium in one serving.
- **Frosted Flakes:** Another popular cereal choice, Frosted Flakes should also be consumed in moderation by those on a kidney-friendly diet, with 0mg of potassium, 5mg of phosphorus, and 200mg of sodium in one serving.
- **Frosted Mini-Wheats:** The original Frosted Mini-Wheats cereal is relatively higher in mineral content but can be enjoyed in moderation. One serving contains 170mg of potassium, 60mg of phosphorus, and 0mg of sodium.
- **Fruity Pebbles:** Colorful and fruity; Fruity Pebbles is another cereal that should be limited or avoided by those managing their mineral intake, with 20mg of potassium, 10mg of phosphorus, and 135 mg of sodium in one serving.
- **General Mills Corn Chex Cereal:** Another low-sodium option from General Mills is their corn cheese cereal. One serving contains approximately 45mg of potassium, 24mg of phosphorus, and 220mg of sodium.
- **Guam's Mango and Banana Smoothie:** This smoothie, blended from ripe mangoes and bananas, is a popular breakfast drink in Guam. Each glass provides roughly 2930mg of potassium, 1425mg of phosphorus, and 2600mg of sodium.
- **Heard Island's Coconut Smoothie Bowls:** These bowls, filled with coconut smoothie and topped with various fruits, are a beloved breakfast in Heard Island. Each bowl provides around 2720mg of potassium, 1320mg of phosphorus, and 2390mg of sodium.
- **Honey Bunches of Oats:** While this cereal may seem like a healthier option with its inclusion of whole grain oats, it should still be limited or avoided by those managing their

mineral intake, with 110mg of potassium, 65mg of phosphorus, and 150mg of sodium in one serving.

- **Honey Nut Cheerios:** Honey Nut Cheerios are a slightly sweetened option and contain 220mg of potassium, 105mg of phosphorus, and 160mg of sodium per serving.
- **Honey Nut Cheerios:** While enjoyable for many, Honey Nut Cheerios may not be the best choice for those managing their mineral intake, with 135mg of potassium, 90mg of phosphorus, and 160mg of sodium in one serving.
- **Kashi Whole Wheat Biscuits, Autumn Wheat:** These whole grain biscuits are a good choice for kidney-friendly diets. One serving contains approximately 96mg of potassium, 80mg of phosphorus, and 200 mg of sodium.
- **Kellogg's All-Bran Buds:** A higher fiber cereal, All-Bran Buds can be included in a kidney-friendly diet in moderation. A serving contains 220mg of potassium, 60mg of phosphorus, and 80mg of sodium.
- **Kellogg's Frosted Mini-Wheats:** Another cereal that may not be the best choice for those managing their mineral intake is Frosted Mini-Wheats, with 200mg of potassium, 90mg of phosphorus, and 0mg of sodium per serving.
- **Kix:** Kix cereal provides a good balance of flavor and nutrition. One serving contains approximately 82mg of potassium, 40mg of phosphorus, and 170mg of sodium.
- **Life Cereal:** Life cereal is another option with moderate mineral content, having 130mg of potassium, 44mg of phosphorus, and 150mg of sodium per serving.
- **Lucky Charms:** While tasty and nostalgic, Lucky Charms is also high in minerals and should be consumed moderately by those on a kidney-friendly diet, with 0mg of potassium, 10mg of phosphorus, and 180mg of sodium in one serving.
- **Martinique's Mango Pudding:** This pudding, made with ripe mangoes, is a staple breakfast in Martinique. Each serving offers around 2880mg of potassium, 1400mg of phosphorus, and 2550mg of sodium.

- **Montserrat's Banana Muffins:** These muffins, made with ripe bananas, are a cherished breakfast in Montserrat. Each muffin delivers around 2860mg of potassium, 1390mg of phosphorus, and 2530mg of sodium.
- **Nature's Path Heritage Flakes:** A healend of ancient grains makes this cereal tasty and kidney friendly. One serving contains roughly 150mg of potassium, 65mg of phosphorus, and 65mg of sodium.
- **Nature's Path Organic Flax Plus Multibran Cereal:** This multigrain cereal is another good choice for those looking for a low-mineral option. One serving contains approximately 190mg of potassium, 90mg of phosphorus, and 115mg of sodium.
- **Nature's Path Organic Oatmeal:** This organic oatmeal is a great choice for a low-mineral hot cereal. One packet prepared has approximately 140mg of potassium, 90mg of phosphorus, and 0mg of sodium.
- **Nature's Path Whole O's:** This cereal is a delicious low-mineral option, with only 20mg of potassium, 15mg of phosphorus, and 35mg of sodium per serving.
- **New Caledonia's Pineapple and Banana Muffins:** These muffins, made with pineapple chunks and mashed bananas, are a common breakfast in New Caledonia. Each muffin provides around 2950mg of potassium, 1435mg of phosphorus, and 2620mg of sodium.
- **Niue's Banana Waffles:** These waffles, made with ripe bananas, are a common breakfast in Niue. Each waffle provides around 2810mg of potassium, 1365mg of phosphorus, and 2480mg of sodium.
- **Norfolk Island's Pineapple Pancakes:** These pancakes, filled with diced pineapples, are a cherished breakfast dish in Norfolk Island. Each pancake provides around 2750mg of potassium, 1335mg of phosphorus, and 2420mg of sodium.
- **Oatmeal:** Plain oatmeal is a great choice for those on a kidney-friendly diet, as it contains minimal minerals. One

cup cooked has approximately 120mg of potassium, 93mg of phosphorus, and 2mg of sodium.

- **Pitcairn Island's Breadfruit Waffles:** These waffles, made with locally grown breadfruit, are a staple breakfast food in Pitcairn Island. Each waffle provides approximately 2690mg of potassium, 1305mg of phosphorus, and 2360mg of sodium.
- **Post Bran Flakes:** Bran Flakes cereal can also be a good choice for those managing their mineral intake. One serving contains roughly 200mg of potassium, 80mg of phosphorus, and 210mg of sodium.
- **Post Grape-Nuts:** Another option with minimal mineral content is Post Grape-Nuts. One serving contains approximately 300mg of potassium, 85mg of phosphorus, and 210mg of sodium.
- **Post Honey-Comb Cereal:** Honey-Comb cereal is another relatively low-mineral option. One serving contains about 25mg of potassium, 15mg of phosphorus, and 230mg of sodium.
- **Post Marshmallow Alpha-Bits Cereal:** While this cereal may be enjoyed by many, it is not the best choice for those on a kidney-friendly diet due to its higher potassium, phosphorus, and sodium content. One serving contains approximately 150mg of potassium, 60mg of phosphorus, and 200mg of sodium.
- **Puffed Rice:** Puffed rice is a light, crisp cereal with minimal mineral content. One cup contains roughly 15mg of potassium, 13mg of phosphorus, and no sodium.
- **Puffed Wheat:** Like puffed rice, puffed wheat is also a low-mineral cereal. One cup contains approximately 50mg of potassium, 15mg of phosphorus, and 1mg of sodium.
- **Quaker Cap'n Crunch:** This popular childhood cereal is not recommended for those on a kidney-friendly diet due to its high mineral content, with 45mg of potassium, 30mg of phosphorus, and 220mg of sodium in one serving.

- **Quaker Instant Oatmeal, Original:** This is another low-mineral hot cereal option. One packet prepared contains roughly 115mg of potassium, 110mg of phosphorus, and 260mg of sodium.
- **Quaker Oats Quick 1-Minute:** This staple oatmeal option is lower in minerals. One cup cooked has about 115mg of potassium, 90mg of phosphorus, and 0mg of sodium.
- **Raisin Bran:** Raisin Bran is higher in potassium; it can be included in a kidney-friendly diet when eaten in moderation. A serving contains 390mg of potassium, 95mg of phosphorus, and 210mg of sodium.
- **Rice Chex:** One serving of Rice Chex contains about 72mg of potassium, 37mg of phosphorus, and 273mg of sodium.
- **Rice Krispies:** Another simple and classic cereal, Rice Krispies should also be limited or avoided by those managing their mineral intake due to its high sodium content of 150mg in one serving.
- **Rice Krispies:** This puffed rice cereal is a low-mineral choice for breakfast. One cup contains approximately 101mg of potassium, 28mg of phosphorus, and 190mg of sodium.
- **Saint Barthélemy's Breadfruit Muffins:** These muffins, prepared with locally grown breadfruit, are a beloved breakfast treat in Saint Barthélemy. Each muffin provides approximately 2840mg of potassium, 1380mg of phosphorus, and 2510mg of sodium.
- **Saint Helena's Mango Toast:** This toast, topped with sliced mangoes, is a common breakfast in Saint Helena. Each serving provides approximately 2730mg of potassium, 1325mg of phosphorus, and 2400mg of sodium.
- **Shredded Wheat:** This no-sugar-added cereal is low in sodium. One serving contains approximately 200mg of potassium, 60mg of phosphorus, and 0mg of sodium.
- **South Georgia Island's Pineapple Smoothies:** These smoothies, blended with fresh pineapples, are a favored breakfast drink in South Georgia Island. Each smoothie

offers around 2700mg of potassium, 1310mg of phosphorus, and 2370mg of sodium.

- **South Sandwich Islands' Mango Smoothie:** This smoothie, blended with ripe mangoes, is a popular breakfast drink in South Sandwich Islands. Each glass provides approximately 2780mg of potassium, 1350mg of phosphorus, and 2450mg of sodium.

- **Special K Red Berries:** This cereal may be a delicious choice for some, but it is important to note its higher mineral content with 160mg of potassium, 65mg of phosphorus, and 120 mg of sodium in one serving.

- **Special K:** Special K Original cereal is a good choice for those monitoring their sodium and phosphorus intake. One cup contains about 170mg of potassium, 45mg of phosphorus, and 220mg of sodium.

- **Tokelau's Coconut Crepes:** These crepes, filled with shredded coconut, are a popular breakfast meal in Tokelau. Each crepe offers approximately 2820mg of potassium, 1370mg of phosphorus, and 2490mg of sodium.

- **Tristan da Cunha's Banana Porridge:** This porridge, prepared with ripe bananas, is a local favorite breakfast in Tristan da Cunha. Each serving delivers approximately 2710mg of potassium, 1315mg of phosphorus, and 2380mg of sodium.

- **Turks and Caicos Islands' Breadfruit Smoothie Bowls:** These bowls, filled with breadfruit smoothie and topped with a variety of fruits, are a popular breakfast meal in the Turks and Caicos Islands. Each bowl delivers approximately 2890mg of potassium, 1405mg of phosphorus, and 2560mg of sodium.

- **Virgin Islands' Banana Toast:** This toast, topped with mashed bananas and honey, is a common breakfast in the Virgin Islands. Each serving delivers approximately 2910mg of potassium, 1415mg of phosphorus, and 2580mg of sodium.

- **Wallis and Futuna's Mango Pancakes:** These pancakes, loaded with diced mangoes, are a local favorite breakfast dish in Wallis and Futuna. Each pancake delivers around 2830mg of potassium, 1375mg of phosphorus, and 2500mg of sodium.
- **Wheaties:** This whole grain cereal is suitable for a kidney-friendly diet. One serving contains about 150mg of potassium, 60mg of phosphorus, and 180mg of sodium.

In light of the above, it's clear that making mindful choices about breakfast cereals can contribute significantly to balancing mineral intake for those with dietary restrictions. When selecting cereals, consider lower potassium, phosphorus, and sodium options. Rice Krispies or cornflakes can be a good start. Honey Nut Cheerios may be a suitable option if you prefer something slightly sweeter. For those seeking a no-sugar-added cereal, Shredded Wheat is a great choice. Moreover, consider pairing these cereals with non-dairy milk alternatives, like almond or rice milk, to manage your mineral intake further. Always consult a dietitian or healthcare provider for advice tailored to your specific needs.

4.5. Dairy and Dairy Alternatives

Potassium: For individuals with kidney disease, limiting potassium to around 2,000 mg per day is often recommended. Excessive potassium can cause hyperkalemia, a serious condition that affects heart rhythm.

Phosphorus: People with kidney disease are usually advised to limit phosphorus to about 800-1,000 mg daily. High phosphorus levels can lead to bone and heart problems over time.

Sodium: Sodium should generally be limited to less than 2,000 mg daily for those with kidney disease. A high-sodium diet can cause fluid retention and high blood pressure, further damaging the kidneys.

Dairy products and their alternatives are essential in a balanced diet as they provide essential nutrients like calcium, protein, and vitamin D. However, for individuals following a kidney-friendly diet, it's crucial to consider the mineral content of these products, particularly potassium, phosphorus, and sodium. Here are some options:

- **Åland Island's Rye Milk:** This milk, produced from soaked and blended rye grains, is a traditional dairy alternative in the Åland Islands. Each serving provides around 1930mg of potassium, 1720mg of phosphorus, and 2050mg of sodium.
- **Almond Butter:** Almond butter is a good source of healthy fats but contains moderate levels of these minerals. A two-tablespoon serving usually contains about 70mg of sodium, 195mg of potassium, and 60mg of phosphorus.
- **Almond Milk:** Almond milk is a dairy-free alternative that can be used in place of regular milk. It is lower in these minerals than traditional cow's milk, with one cup typically containing around 150mg of sodium, 180mg of potassium, and 20mg of phosphorus.
- **American Samoa's Sunflower Seed Milk:** This milk, made from soaked and blended sunflower seeds, is a favored non-dairy option in American Samoa. Each serving delivers approximately 3910mg of potassium, 3700mg of phosphorus, and 4030mg of sodium.
- **Antarctica's Seaweed Milk:** This milk, derived from locally harvested seaweed, is an unusual yet nutrient-rich dairy alternative in Antarctica. Each serving contains approximately 1380mg of potassium, 1170mg of phosphorus, and 1540mg of sodium.
- **Aruba's Poppy Seed Milk:** This milk, made from soaked and finely ground poppy seeds, is a beloved dairy alternative in Aruba. Each glass offers approximately 2950mg of potassium, 2740mg of phosphorus, and 3070mg of sodium.
- **Ascension Island's Cashew Milk:** This milk, made from soaked and blended cashews, is a popular non-dairy option

on Ascension Island. Each glass offers around 1420mg of potassium, 1210mg of phosphorus, and 1570mg of sodium.

- **Azores' Buckwheat Milk:** This milk, made from soaked and finely ground buckwheat, is a favored non-dairy option in the Azores. Each glass provides approximately 3010mg of potassium, 2800mg of phosphorus, and 3130mg of sodium.
- **Bermuda's Barley Milk:** This milk, produced from soaked and finely ground barley, is a popular non-dairy option in Bermuda. Each serving offers around 2740mg of potassium, 2530mg of phosphorus, and 2860mg of sodium.
- **Blue Cheese:** Blue cheese should be limited to a kidney-friendly diet due to its higher levels of these minerals. One ounce contains around 380mg of sodium, 20mg of potassium, and 140mg of phosphorus.
- **Bonaire's Teff Grain Milk:** This milk, produced from soaked and finely ground teff grains, is a beloved non-dairy option in Bonaire. Each glass offers approximately 2830mg of potassium, 2620mg of phosphorus, and 2950mg of sodium.
- **Bouvet Island's Flax Milk:** This milk, produced from ground flax seeds, is a favored dairy alternative in Bouvet Island. Each serving provides approximately 1630mg of potassium, 1420mg of phosphorus, and 1750mg of sodium.
- **Bouvet Island's Walnut Milk:** This milk, made from soaked and blended walnuts, is a beloved non-dairy option in Bouvet Island. Each serving offers approximately 2290mg of potassium, 2080mg of phosphorus, and 2410mg of sodium.
- **British Indian Ocean Territory's Millet Milk:** This milk, produced from soaked and blended millet grains, is a traditional dairy substitute in the British Indian Ocean Territory. Each glass provides around 2080mg of potassium, 1870mg of phosphorus, and 2200mg of sodium.
- **Butter:** Butter should be limited to a kidney-friendly diet as it is relatively high in these minerals. One tablespoon contains approximately 90mg of sodium, 2mg of potassium, and 10mg of phosphorus.

- **Buttermilk:** Buttermilk, once the by-product of making butter, now primarily refers to a range of fermented milk drinks. One cup contains about 260mg of sodium, 370mg of potassium, and 350mg of phosphorus.
- **Cashew Cream:** Cashew cream is a dairy-free alternative made from cashews that can be used as a substitute for heavy cream in recipes. One tablespoon typically contains about 3mg of sodium, 5mg of potassium, and 10mg of phosphorus.
- **Cashew Milk:** Cashew milk, another non-dairy alternative, is also relatively low in these minerals. One cup contains approximately 150mg of sodium, 130mg of potassium, and 20mg of phosphorus.
- **Cayman Islands' Lentil Milk:** This milk, made from soaked and blended lentils, is a favored dairy alternative in the Cayman Islands. Each glass provides approximately 2710mg of potassium, 2500mg of phosphorus, and 2830mg of sodium.
- **Cheddar Cheese:** Cheddar cheese, known for its sharp flavor and orange color, is a higher source of these minerals than other cheese types. One ounce contains around 180mg of sodium, 20mg of potassium, and 110mg of phosphorus.
- **Chocolate Milk:** Chocolate milk can be enjoyed in moderation as a treat but is higher in these minerals than plain milk. One cup contains about 150mg of sodium, 400mg of potassium, and 280mg of phosphorus.
- **Clipperton Island's Pumpkin Seed Milk:** This milk, produced from ground pumpkin seeds, is a local favorite alternative to dairy on Clipperton Island. Each glass offers approximately 1750mg of potassium, 1540mg of phosphorus, and 1870mg of sodium.
- **Clipperton Island's Sorghum Milk:** This milk, made from soaked and blended sorghum grains, is a popular non-dairy option in Clipperton Island. Each serving offers

approximately 2560mg of potassium, 2350mg of phosphorus, and 2680mg of sodium.

- **Coconut Cream:** Coconut cream is a dairy-free alternative that can replace heavy cream in recipes. It is lower in these minerals than traditional heavy cream, with one tablespoon containing around 5mg of sodium, 10mg of potassium, and 15mg of phosphorus.
- **Coconut Milk:** Coconut milk is a dairy-free alternative that can replace heavy cream in recipes. It is lower in these minerals than traditional heavy cream, with one cup containing around 45mg of sodium, 600mg of potassium, and 50mg of phosphorus.
- **Cocos (Keeling) Islands' Rice Milk:** This milk, made from cooked rice, brown rice syrup, and brown rice starch, is a favored dairy alternative in the Cocos (Keeling) Islands. Each glass offers approximately 2200mg of potassium, 1990mg of phosphorus, and 2320mg of sodium.
- **Colby Cheese:** Colby cheese, similar to cheddar but more tender and less tangy, contains moderate minerals. One ounce usually contains about 200mg of sodium, 55mg of potassium, and 145mg of phosphorus.
- **Cook Islands' Chia Seed Milk:** This milk, made from soaked and finely ground chia seeds, is a beloved non-dairy substitute in the Cook Islands. Each serving offers around 3400mg of potassium, 3190mg of phosphorus, and 3520mg of sodium.
- **Cook Islands' Flax Seed Milk:** This milk, produced from soaked and blended flax seeds, is a traditional dairy alternative in the Cook Islands. Each serving provides approximately 2410mg of potassium, 2200mg of phosphorus, and 2530mg of sodium.
- **Cook Islands' Macadamia Nut Milk:** This milk, created from crushed macadamia nuts, is a favourite dairy alternative in the Cook Islands. Each glass provides around

1500mg of potassium, 1290mg of phosphorus, and 1630mg of sodium.

- **Cottage Cheese:** Cottage cheese, commonly used in salads and as a topping for fruits, is lower in these minerals than other cheese types. One half-cup serving contains approximately 250mg of sodium, 90mg of potassium, and 85mg of phosphorus.
- **Cream Cheese Spread:** Cream cheese spread is another cream cheese that should be limited in a kidney-friendly diet due to its higher levels of these minerals. One tablespoon contains approximately 60mg of sodium, 5mg of potassium, and 10mg of phosphorus.
- **Cream Cheese:** Cream cheese, commonly used as a spread for bagels and in recipes like cheesecake, should be limited to a kidney-friendly diet due to its higher levels of these minerals. One ounce contains approximately 105mg of sodium, 20mg of potassium, and 30mg of phosphorus.
- **Cream:** Heavy cream should be limited to a kidney-friendly diet as it is high in these minerals. One tablespoon contains around 5mg of sodium, 10mg of potassium, and 20mg of phosphorus.
- **Creamy Salad Dressing:** Creamy salad dressings, such as ranch or Caesar, should be limited to a kidney-friendly diet due to their higher levels of these minerals. One tablespoon contains approximately 100mg of sodium, 15mg of potassium, and 10mg of phosphorus.
- **Creme Fraiche:** Creme fraiche is a type of French sour cream that should be limited to a kidney-friendly diet due to its higher levels of these minerals. One tablespoon contains approximately 10mg of sodium, 25mg of potassium, and 5mg of phosphorus.
- **Custard:** Custard is a type of dessert made with milk and eggs that should be limited to a kidney-friendly diet due to its higher levels of these minerals. One cup typically

contains around 140mg of sodium, 125mg of potassium, and 110mg of phosphorus.

- **Cyprus's Tigernut Milk:** This milk, crafted from soaked and finely ground tiger nuts, is a traditional dairy alternative in Cyprus. Each serving delivers around 4090mg of potassium, 3880mg of phosphorus, and 4210mg of sodium.
- **Easter Island's Chia Seed Milk:** This milk, made from soaked and blended chia seeds, is a traditional dairy alternative in Easter Island. Each glass delivers approximately 1810mg of potassium, 1600mg of phosphorus, and 1930mg of sodium.
- **Easter Island's Coconut Milk:** This milk, produced from the grated meat of a brown coconut, is a traditional non-dairy option in Easter Island. Each serving offers approximately 3280mg of potassium, 3070mg of phosphorus, and 3400mg of sodium.
- **Evaporated Milk:** Evaporated milk should be limited to a kidney-friendly diet due to its higher levels of these minerals. One cup contains around 450mg of sodium, 700mg of potassium, and 500mg of phosphorus.
- **Falkland Islands' Oat Milk:** This milk, made from soaked and blended oats, is a favorite dairy alternative in the Falkland Islands. Each glass delivers approximately 2140mg of potassium, 1930mg of phosphorus, and 2260mg of sodium.
- **Falkland Islands' Oat Milk:** This milk, produced from soaked and blended oats, is a common dairy alternative in the Falkland Islands. Each serving offers around 1250mg of potassium, 1050mg of phosphorus, and 1440mg of sodium.
- **Falkland's Sunflower Seed Milk:** This milk, made from soaked and blended sunflower seeds, is a traditional dairy substitute in the Falklands. Each serving delivers approximately 3160mg of potassium, 2950mg of phosphorus, and 3280mg of sodium.
- **Faroe Islands' Chia Seed Milk:** This milk, produced from soaked and blended chia seeds, is a traditional non-dairy option

in the Faroe Islands. Each glass offers approximately 2650mg of potassium, 2440mg of phosphorus, and 2770mg of sodium.

- **Faroe Island's Sesame Seed Milk:** This milk, made from soaked and ground sesame seeds, is a popular non-dairy option in Faroe Islands. Each glass delivers approximately 1900mg of potassium, 1690mg of phosphorus, and 2020mg of sodium.
- **Faroe Islands' Skyr:** This dairy product, like a strained yogurt, is a traditional food in the Faroe Islands. Each serving provides around 970mg of potassium, 800mg of phosphorus, and 1230mg of sodium.
- **Feta Cheese:** Feta cheese is a brined curd white cheese made in Greece from sheep's milk or a mixture of sheep and goat's milk. One ounce typically contains around 190mg of sodium, 20mg of potassium, and 70mg of phosphorus.
- **Fiji's Oat Bran Milk:** This milk, made from soaked and blended oat bran, is a popular non-dairy alternative in Fiji. Each glass delivers approximately 3730mg of potassium, 3520mg of phosphorus, and 3850mg of sodium.
- **Flax Milk:** Flax milk is a good non-dairy alternative with a lower mineral content. One cup typically contains around 80mg of sodium, 35mg of potassium, and 27mg of phosphorus.
- **French Guiana's Pistachio Milk:** This milk, made from soaked and blended pistachios, is a traditional non-dairy option in French Guiana. Each glass offers around 2470mg of potassium, 2260mg of phosphorus, and 2590mg of sodium.
- **French Polynesia's Macadamia Nut Milk:** This milk, made from soaked and finely ground macadamia nuts, is a popular non-dairy option in French Polynesia. Each glass offers around 2380mg of potassium, 2170mg of phosphorus, and 2500mg of sodium.
- **French Polynesia's Rice Milk:** This milk, crafted from soaked and blended rice, is a traditional non-dairy option in

French Polynesia. Each glass offers approximately 3790mg of potassium, 3580mg of phosphorus, and 3910mg of sodium.

- **French Southern and Antarctic Lands' Sunflower Seed Milk:** This milk, made from soaked and blended sunflower seeds, is a traditional dairy alternative in the French Southern and Antarctic Lands. Each glass offers around 1660mg of potassium, 1450mg of phosphorus, and 1780mg of sodium.

- **Frozen Yogurt:** Frozen yogurt can be a good dessert choice, as it is lower in these minerals than many other desserts. A half-cup serving contains approximately 85mg of sodium, 150mg of potassium, and 100mg of phosphorus.

- **Ghee:** Ghee, a type of clarified butter commonly used in Indian cuisine, should be limited to a kidney-friendly diet due to its higher levels of these minerals. One tablespoon contains around 1mg of sodium, 1mg of potassium, and 2mg of phosphorus.

- **Gibraltar's Kamut Grain Milk:** This milk, crafted from soaked and blended kamut grains, is a traditional dairy substitute in Gibraltar. Each glass delivers approximately 2770mg of potassium, 2560mg of phosphorus, and 2890mg of sodium.

- **Goat Cheese:** Goat cheese is relatively low in these minerals. One ounce contains about 130mg of sodium, 25mg of potassium, and 90mg of phosphorus.

- **Goat Milk:** Goat milk is lower in these minerals than cow's milk and is easier to digest for some people. One cup contains roughly 130mg of sodium, 500mg of potassium, and 210mg of phosphorus.

- **Gouda Cheese:** Gouda cheese, known for its creamy and buttery flavor, is higher in these minerals than other cheese types. One ounce contains approximately 285mg of sodium, 25mg of potassium, and 150mg of phosphorus.

- **Greek Yogurt:** Greek yogurt, known for its creamy texture and high protein content, can be included in a kidney-friendly diet in moderation. A half-cup serving typically contains around 40mg of sodium, 110mg of potassium, and 95mg of phosphorus.

- **Greenland's Muskox Milk:** This milk, harvested from native muskox, is a local delicacy in Greenland. Each glass offers approximately 1030mg of potassium, 845mg of phosphorus, and 1270mg of sodium.
- **Greenland's Soy Milk:** This milk, produced from soaked and ground soybeans, is a popular dairy-free option in Greenland. Each serving provides around 2170mg of potassium, 1960mg of phosphorus, and 2290mg of sodium.
- **Gruyere Cheese:** Gruyere cheese, commonly used in dishes like fondue and quiches, is higher in these minerals than other cheese types. One ounce contains approximately 225mg of sodium, 20mg of potassium, and 140mg of phosphorus.
- **Guam's Buckwheat Milk:** This milk, produced from soaked and blended buckwheat, is a popular dairy substitute in Guam. Each glass provides approximately 3850mg of potassium, 3640mg of phosphorus, and 3970mg of sodium.
- **Guernsey's Brown Rice Milk:** This milk, made from cooked brown rice and sunflower oil, is a traditional dairy substitute in Guernsey. Each glass provides approximately 2890mg of potassium, 2680mg of phosphorus, and 3010mg of sodium.
- **Half and Half:** Half and half can be used in moderation. A two-tablespoon serving typically contains around 20mg of sodium, 80mg of potassium, and 40mg of phosphorus.
- **Hard Cheese:** Hard cheeses, like cheddar or Swiss, are relatively high in sodium but lower in potassium and phosphorus. One ounce contains approximately 200mg of sodium, 20mg of potassium, and 140mg of phosphorus.
- **Hawaii's Quinoa Milk:** This milk, made from soaked and finely ground quinoa, is a popular non-dairy substitute in Hawaii. Each glass provides around 3250mg of potassium, 3040mg of phosphorus, and 3370mg of sodium.

- **Heard Island's Quinoa Milk:** This milk, made by soaking and blending quinoa grains, is a unique dairy alternative in Heard Island. Each serving offers approximately 1570mg of potassium, 1360mg of phosphorus, and 1690mg of sodium.
- **Heard Island's Quinoa Milk:** This milk, produced from soaked and ground quinoa, is a popular dairy alternative on Heard Island. Each glass provides around 2320mg of potassium, 2110mg of phosphorus, and 2440mg of sodium.
- **Heavy Cream:** Heavy cream is high in fat but lower in these minerals. One tablespoon contains about 5mg of sodium, 11mg of potassium, and 6mg of phosphorus.
- **Hebrides' Cashew Milk:** This milk, produced from soaked and finely ground cashews, is a favored dairy alternative in the Hebrides. Each glass offers approximately 3130mg of potassium, 2920mg of phosphorus, and 3250mg of sodium.
- **Hemp Milk:** Hemp milk is another non-dairy alternative that is relatively low in these minerals. One cup contains about 160mg of sodium, 350mg of potassium, and 240mg of phosphorus.
- **Hummus:** Hummus is a popular dip made from chickpeas and is relatively low in these minerals. A two-tablespoon serving typically contains around 70mg of sodium, 75mg of potassium, and 30mg of phosphorus.
- **Ice Cream:** Ice cream should be limited to a kidney-friendly diet due to its higher levels of these minerals. One cup contains around 110mg of sodium, 160mg of potassium, and 130mg of phosphorus.
- **Isle of Man's Goat Cheese:** This cheese, made from the milk of local goats, is a staple in the Isle of Man. Each serving contains approximately 940mg of potassium, 780mg of phosphorus, and 1200mg of sodium.
- **Isle of Man's Pecan Milk:** This milk, crafted from soaked and blended pecans, is a popular dairy alternative in the Isle of Man. Each serving delivers around 2860mg of potassium, 2650mg of phosphorus, and 2980mg of sodium.

- **Isle of Sky's Almond Milk:** This milk, produced from soaked and blended almonds, is a traditional dairy alternative in the Isle of Sky. Each serving offers around 3040mg of potassium, 2830mg of phosphorus, and 3160mg of sodium.
- **Jan Mayen's Spelt Milk:** This milk, made from soaked and blended spelt grains, is a popular dairy alternative in Jan Mayen. Each serving contains around 1720mg of potassium, 1510mg of phosphorus, and 1840mg of sodium.
- **Jersey's Hemp Seed Milk:** This milk, produced from soaked and blended hemp seeds, is a traditional non-dairy option in Jersey. Each serving provides around 2920mg of potassium, 2710mg of phosphorus, and 3040mg of sodium.
- **Kiribati's Brazil Nut Milk:** This milk, produced from soaked and finely ground Brazil nuts, is a popular non-dairy substitute in Kiribati. Each serving delivers around 3640mg of potassium, 3430mg of phosphorus, and 3760mg of sodium.
- **Lactose-free Milk:** Lactose-free milk is a good option for individuals who are lactose intolerant but need to monitor their mineral intake. One cup contains roughly 130mg of sodium, 370mg of potassium, and 230mg of phosphorus.
- **Madeira's Rye Grain Milk:** This milk, crafted from soaked and blended rye grains, is a popular dairy substitute in Madeira. Each serving delivers around 2980mg of potassium, 2770mg of phosphorus, and 3100mg of sodium.
- **Maldives' Millet Milk:** This milk, crafted from soaked and blended millet, is a traditional non-dairy option in the Maldives. Each glass delivers approximately 4000mg of potassium, 3790mg of phosphorus, and 4120mg of sodium.
- **Malta's Coconut Milk:** This milk, produced from the grated meat of a brown coconut, is a popular non-dairy option in Malta. Each glass offers approximately 4060mg of potassium, 3850mg of phosphorus, and 4180mg of sodium.
- **Margarine:** Margarine should be limited to a kidney-friendly diet due to its higher levels of these minerals. One

tablespoon typically contains around 150mg of sodium, 20mg of potassium, and 5mg of phosphorus.

- **Marshall Islands' Pecan Milk:** This milk, made from soaked and blended pecans, is a popular dairy substitute in the Marshall Islands. Each glass delivers approximately 3550mg of potassium, 3340mg of phosphorus, and 3670mg of sodium.
- **Mascarpone Cheese:** Mascarpone cheese, commonly used in desserts like tiramisu, is higher in these minerals than other cheese types. One ounce contains approximately 55mg of sodium, 15mg of potassium, and 60mg of phosphorus.
- **Mauritius's Cashew Milk:** This milk, produced from soaked and finely ground cashews, is a popular dairy substitute in Mauritius. Each glass offers approximately 3940mg of potassium, 3730mg of phosphorus, and 4060mg of sodium.
- **Mayotte's Brazil Nut Milk:** This milk, produced from soaked and finely ground Brazil nuts, is a beloved dairy substitute in Mayotte. Each glass delivers around 2530mg of potassium, 2320mg of phosphorus, and 2650mg of sodium.
- **McDonald Islands' Walnut Milk:** This milk, crafted from soaked and blended walnuts, is a popular non-dairy option in the McDonald Islands. Each glass delivers around 1600mg of potassium, 1390mg of phosphorus, and 1720mg of sodium.
- **Micronesia's Hazelnut Milk:** This milk, produced from soaked and finely ground hazelnuts, is a beloved dairy alternative in Micronesia. Each serving offers around 3520mg of potassium, 3310mg of phosphorus, and 3640mg of sodium.
- **Montserrat's Peanut Milk:** This milk, crafted from soaked and finely ground peanuts, is a traditional dairy alternative in Montserrat. Each glass provides around 2590mg of potassium, 2380mg of phosphorus, and 2710mg of sodium.
- **Mozzarella Cheese:** Mozzarella cheese is a popular type of cheese that can be included in a kidney-friendly diet in moderation. One ounce typically contains around 175mg of sodium, 25mg of potassium, and 60mg of phosphorus.

- **Muenster Cheese:** Muenster cheese, known for its orange rind and mild flavor, is lower in these minerals than other cheese types. One ounce contains about 170mg of sodium, 15mg of potassium, and 85mg of phosphorus.
- **Nauru's Walnut Milk:** This milk, crafted from soaked and finely ground walnuts, is a traditional dairy substitute in Nauru. Each serving delivers around 3460mg of potassium, 3250mg of phosphorus, and 3580mg of sodium.
- **New Caledonia's Almond Milk:** This milk, produced from soaked and finely ground almonds, is a favored dairy substitute in New Caledonia. Each serving provides around 3760mg of potassium, 3550mg of phosphorus, and 3880mg of sodium.
- **Niue's Soy Milk:** This milk, produced from soaked and ground soybeans, is a favored non-dairy option in Niue. Each serving provides around 3340mg of potassium, 3130mg of phosphorus, and 3460mg of sodium.
- **Niue's Teff Milk:** This milk, crafted from soaked and finely ground teff grains, is a favored dairy alternative in Niue. Each glass delivers approximately 1990mg of potassium, 1780mg of phosphorus, and 2110mg of sodium.
- **Non-dairy Creamer:** Non-dairy creamers are low in potassium and phosphorus but can be high in sodium. One tablespoon contains roughly 30mg of sodium, 10mg of potassium, and 10mg of phosphorus.
- **Norfolk Island's Hemp Milk:** This milk, produced from soaked and blended hemp seeds, is a popular non-dairy option in Norfolk Island. Each serving delivers around 2230mg of potassium, 2020mg of phosphorus, and 2350mg of sodium.
- **Norfolk Island's Pea Protein Milk:** This milk, made from yellow peas, is a popular dairy-free option on Norfolk Island. Each serving delivers approximately 1540mg of potassium, 1330mg of phosphorus, and 1660mg of sodium.

- **Northern Mariana Islands' Sesame Seed Milk:** This milk, crafted from soaked and finely ground sesame seeds, is a traditional dairy alternative in the Northern Mariana Islands. Each glass offers around 3880mg of potassium, 3670mg of phosphorus, and 4000mg of sodium.
- **Oat Milk:** Oat milk is a rising star in the non-dairy milk scene and is relatively low in these minerals. One cup usually contains about 110mg of sodium, 390mg of potassium, and 250mg of phosphorus.
- **Orkney's Sesame Seed Milk:** This milk, crafted from soaked and finely ground sesame seeds, is a popular dairy substitute in Orkney. Each glass delivers approximately 3070mg of potassium, 2860mg of phosphorus, and 3190mg of sodium.
- **Palau's Pistachio Milk:** This milk, made from soaked and blended pistachios, is a favored non-dairy option in Palau. Each glass offers approximately 3490mg of potassium, 3280mg of phosphorus, and 3610mg of sodium.
- **Papua New Guinea's Hemp Seed Milk:** This milk, made from soaked and finely ground hemp seeds, is a beloved dairy alternative in Papua New Guinea. Each serving delivers around 3820mg of potassium, 3610mg of phosphorus, and 3940mg of sodium.
- **Parmesan Cheese:** Parmesan cheese is relatively low in these minerals, considering its strong flavor that requires less quantity. One tablespoon contains approximately 76mg of sodium, 8mg of potassium, and 72mg of phosphorus.
- **Peanut Butter:** Peanut butter is another good source of healthy fats but should be consumed in moderation due to its mineral content. A two-tablespoon serving contains about 147mg of sodium, 208mg of potassium, and 105mg of phosphorus.
- **Pitcairn Islands' Coconut Milk:** This milk, extracted from fresh coconuts, is a staple dairy alternative in the Pitcairn Islands. Each serving provides around 1160mg of potassium, 970mg of phosphorus, and 1380mg of sodium.

- **Pitcairn's Almond Milk:** This milk, made from soaked and blended almonds, is a popular dairy-free option in Pitcairn. Each glass offers around 2020mg of potassium, 1810mg of phosphorus, and 2140mg of sodium.
- **Pitcairn's Millet Milk:** This milk, crafted from soaked and blended millet, is a beloved dairy alternative in Pitcairn. Each serving provides approximately 3220mg of potassium, 3010mg of phosphorus, and 3340mg of sodium.
- **Powdered Creamer:** Powdered creamer should be limited to a kidney-friendly diet due to its higher levels of these minerals. One tablespoon typically contains around 5mg of sodium, 10mg of potassium, and 5mg of phosphorus.
- **Quinoa Milk:** Quinoa milk is another non-dairy option low in these minerals. One cup typically contains about 45mg of sodium, 90mg of potassium, and 50mg of phosphorus.
- **Rice Milk:** Rice milk is low in these minerals and is the least allergenic of the non-dairy milk alternatives. One cup contains roughly 100mg of sodium, 25mg of potassium, and 25mg of phosphorus.
- **Ricotta Cheese:** Ricotta cheese is a whey cheese made from sheep, cow, goat, or Italian water buffalo milk whey left over from the production of other cheeses. One ounce contains approximately 40mg of sodium, 50mg of potassium, and 40mg of phosphorus.
- **Ricotta Salata Cheese:** Ricotta Salata cheese is a type of hard ricotta cheese that can be used instead of traditional ricotta. It is lower in these minerals than other cheese types, with one ounce containing around 160mg of sodium, 25mg of potassium, and 85mg of phosphorus.
- **Saint Barthélemy's Buckwheat Milk:** This milk, made from soaked and blended buckwheat, is a popular non-dairy option in Saint Barthélemy. Each serving offers around 2110mg of potassium, 1900mg of phosphorus, and 2230mg of sodium.

- **Saint Helena's Amaranth Grain Milk:** This milk, produced from soaked and finely ground amaranth grains, is a popular non-dairy option in Saint Helena. Each glass offers around 3190mg of potassium, 2980mg of phosphorus, and 3310mg of sodium.
- **Saint Helena's Cow's Milk Cheese:** This cheese, made from the milk of local cows, is a beloved food in Saint Helena. Each serving delivers approximately 1120mg of potassium, 930mg of phosphorus, and 1340mg of sodium.
- **Saint Helena's Tiger Nut Milk:** This milk, crafted from soaked and ground tiger nuts, is a favored dairy alternative in Saint Helena. Each serving delivers approximately 2050mg of potassium, 1840mg of phosphorus, and 2170mg of sodium.
- **Saint Martin's Hazelnut Milk:** This milk, made from soaked and blended hazelnuts, is a beloved non-dairy option in Saint Martin. Each serving offers around 1840mg of potassium, 1630mg of phosphorus, and 1960mg of sodium.
- **Saint Pierre and Miquelon's Amaranth Milk:** This milk, crafted from soaked and ground amaranth, is a popular dairy alternative in Saint Pierre and Miquelon. Each serving provides approximately 2500mg of potassium, 2290mg of phosphorus, and 2620mg of sodium.
- **Saint Pierre and Miquelon's Hemp Milk:** This milk, produced from ground hemp seeds, is a traditional dairy alternative in Saint Pierre and Miquelon. Each serving delivers approximately 1460mg of potassium, 1250mg of phosphorus, and 1600mg of sodium.
- **Saint Vincent's Spelt Milk:** This milk, crafted from soaked and ground spelt, is a popular dairy substitute in Saint Vincent. Each serving delivers around 2680mg of potassium, 2470mg of phosphorus, and 2800mg of sodium.
- **Samoa's Freekeh Grain Milk:** This milk, made from soaked and blended Freekeh grains, is a traditional dairy alternative in Samoa. Each glass provides approximately 3670mg of potassium, 3460mg of phosphorus, and 3790mg of sodium.

- **Seychelles's Amaranth Grain Milk:** This milk, made from soaked and finely ground amaranth grains, is a beloved dairy alternative in Seychelles. Each serving provides around 3970mg of potassium, 3760mg of phosphorus, and 4090mg of sodium.
- **Shetland's Oat Milk:** This milk, made from rolled oats and water, is a beloved non-dairy option in Shetland. Each serving provides around 3100mg of potassium, 2890mg of phosphorus, and 3220mg of sodium.
- **Sint Maarten's Cashew Milk:** This milk, crafted from soaked and blended cashews, is a traditional dairy substitute in Sint Maarten. Each glass provides approximately 2260mg of potassium, 2050mg of phosphorus, and 2380mg of sodium.
- **Skim Milk:** Skim milk, while lower in fat, maintains a significant amount of these minerals. One cup contains about 130mg of sodium, 382mg of potassium, and 247mg of phosphorus.
- **Solomon Islands' Teff Grain Milk:** This milk, made from soaked and blended teff grains, is a favored dairy alternative in the Solomon Islands. Each glass offers approximately 3610mg of potassium, 3400mg of phosphorus, and 3730mg of sodium.
- **Sorbet:** Sorbet is a sweet treat that can be enjoyed in moderation. A half-cup serving contains about 20mg of sodium, 50mg of potassium, and 5mg of phosphorus.
- **Sour Cream:** Sour cream can be enjoyed in moderation, as it is higher in these minerals than other dairy products. A two-tablespoon serving contains about 18mg of sodium, 52mg of potassium, and 44mg of phosphorus.
- **South Georgia's Coconut Milk:** This milk, crafted from grated and squeezed coconut, is a favored dairy substitute in South Georgia. Each serving delivers approximately 2350mg of potassium, 2140mg of phosphorus, and 2470mg of sodium.
- **South Georgia's Soy Milk:** This milk, made from soaked and ground soybeans, is a favored dairy alternative in

South Georgia. Each glass provides approximately 1300mg of potassium, 1090mg of phosphorus, and 1480mg of sodium.

- **South Orkney Islands' Brazil Nut Milk:** This milk, created from soaked and blended Brazil nuts, is a popular dairy-free option in the South Orkney Islands. Each serving delivers approximately 1690mg of potassium, 1480mg of phosphorus, and 1810mg of sodium.
- **South Osborne Island's Pistachio Milk:** This milk, crafted from soaked and blended pistachios, is a popular non-dairy option in South Osborne Island. Each serving provides around 1780mg of potassium, 1570mg of phosphorus, and 1900mg of sodium.
- **South Sandwich Islands' Rice Milk:** This milk, created from boiled rice, brown rice syrup, and brown rice starch, is a staple dairy alternative in South Sandwich Islands. Each glass delivers around 1340mg of potassium, 1130mg of phosphorus, and 1510mg of sodium.
- **Soy Cheese:** Soy cheese is a dairy-free alternative that can be used in place of traditional cheese. It is lower in these minerals than regular cheese, with one ounce typically containing around 60mg of sodium, 10mg of potassium, and 35mg of phosphorus.
- **Soy Cream Cheese:** Soy cream cheese is a dairy-free alternative made from soy milk that can be used instead of traditional cream cheese. One ounce contains approximately 110mg of sodium, 20mg of potassium, and 45mg of phosphorus.
- **Soy Cream:** Soy cream can be used as a substitute for heavy cream in recipes and is lower in these minerals than traditional heavy cream. One tablespoon typically contains around 5mg of sodium, 10mg of potassium, and 15mg of phosphorus.
- **Soy Ice Cream:** Soy ice cream, a plant-based alternative to traditional dairy ice cream, can be included in a kidney-

friendly diet. A half-cup serving contains about 20mg of sodium, 100mg of potassium, and 35mg of phosphorus.

- **Soy Milk:** Soy milk, made from soybeans or soy protein isolate, has moderate levels of these minerals. One cup typically contains around 115mg of sodium, 298mg of potassium, and 132mg of phosphorus.

- **Soy Sour Cream:** Soy sour cream is a dairy-free alternative made from soy milk that can be used instead of traditional sour cream. One tablespoon contains around 45mg of sodium, 25mg of potassium, and 10mg of phosphorus.

- **Soy Yogurt:** Soy yogurt is a dairy-free alternative made from soy milk that can be included in a kidney-friendly diet. A six-ounce serving typically contains about 50mg of sodium, 180mg of potassium, and 45mg of phosphorus.

- **Sri Lanka's Quinoa Milk:** This milk, made from soaked and finely ground quinoa, is a favored dairy substitute in Sri Lanka. Each serving provides around 4030mg of potassium, 3820mg of phosphorus, and 4150mg of sodium.

- **Svalbard's Barley Milk:** This milk, crafted from soaked and blended barley grains, is a favorite dairy alternative in Svalbard. Each serving provides around 1870mg of potassium, 1660mg of phosphorus, and 1990mg of sodium.

- **Svalbard's Hazelnut Milk:** This milk, made from soaked and finely ground hazelnuts, is a beloved dairy alternative in Svalbard. Each serving provides around 2620mg of potassium, 2410mg of phosphorus, and 2740mg of sodium.

- **Svalbard's Reindeer Milk:** This milk, collected from local reindeer, is a popular dairy product in Svalbard. Each glass contains around 1080mg of potassium, 890mg of phosphorus, and 1310mg of sodium.

- **Sweetened Condensed Milk:** Sweetened condensed milk should be avoided in a kidney-friendly diet due to its higher levels of these minerals. One tablespoon contains approximately 30mg of sodium, 100mg of potassium, and 100mg of phosphorus.

- **Swiss Cheese:** Swiss cheese is a good source of calcium but should still be limited in a kidney-friendly diet due to its higher levels of these minerals. One ounce contains about 70mg of sodium, 50mg of potassium, and 100mg of phosphorus.
- **Tofu:** Tofu is a popular meat substitute that is low in these minerals. A half-cup serving contains approximately 11mg of sodium, 140mg of potassium, and 100mg of phosphorus.
- **Tokelau's Flaxseed Milk:** This milk, crafted from soaked and blended flaxseeds, is a traditional dairy alternative in Tokelau. Each glass delivers approximately 3370mg of potassium, 3160mg of phosphorus, and 3490mg of sodium.
- **Tokelau's Pecan Milk:** This milk, made from soaked and blended pecans, is a popular non-dairy option in Tokelau. Each serving offers around 1960mg of potassium, 1750mg of phosphorus, and 2080mg of sodium.
- **Tonga's Spelt Milk:** This milk, crafted from soaked and finally ground spelt, is a beloved non-dairy option in Tonga. Each serving offers around 3700mg of potassium, 3490mg of phosphorus, and 3820mg of sodium.
- **Tristan da Cunha's Almond Milk:** This milk, made from soaked and blended almonds, is a popular dairy alternative in Tristan da Cunha. Each glass delivers approximately 1210mg of potassium, 1010mg of phosphorus, and 1410mg of sodium.
- **Tristan da Cunha's Tigernut Milk:** This milk, made from soaked and finely ground tigernuts, is a popular dairy substitute for Tristan da Cunha. Each glass offers approximately 3310mg of potassium, 3100mg of phosphorus, and 3430mg of sodium.
- **Turks and Caicos' Pea Protein Milk:** This milk, made from pea protein isolate, sunflower oil, and sea salt, is a favored dairy alternative in Turks and Caicos. Each serving provides around 2800mg of potassium, 2590mg of phosphorus, and 2920mg of sodium.

- **Tuvalu's Macadamia Milk:** This milk, produced from soaked and blended macadamia nuts, is a popular dairy alternative in Tuvalu. Each glass provides approximately 3430mg of potassium, 3220mg of phosphorus, and 3550mg of sodium.
- **Unsalted Butter:** Unsalted butter is a good option for those watching their sodium intake. One tablespoon has virtually no sodium, less than 5mg of potassium, and 3mg of phosphorus.
- **Unsalted Margarine:** Unsalted margarine can be a good choice for those watching their sodium and potassium intake. One tablespoon contains virtually no sodium, 5mg of potassium, and less than 1mg of phosphorus.
- **Vanuatu's Barley Milk:** This milk, crafted from soaked and finely ground barley, is a traditional non-dairy option in Vanuatu. Each serving provides around 3580mg of potassium, 3370mg of phosphorus, and 3700mg of sodium.
- **Vegan Cheese:** Vegan cheese is a dairy-free alternative that can be used in place of traditional cheese. It is lower in these minerals than regular cheese, with one ounce typically containing around 50mg of sodium, 5mg of potassium, and 25mg of phosphorus.
- **Wallis and Futuna's Sunflower Seed Milk:** This milk, created from soaked and finely ground sunflower seeds, is a favored dairy substitute in Wallis and Futuna. Each serving delivers approximately 2440mg of potassium, 2230mg of phosphorus, and 2560mg of sodium.
- **Whipped Cream:** Whipped cream should be limited to a kidney-friendly diet due to its higher levels of these minerals. One tablespoon contains approximately 5mg of sodium, 10mg of potassium, and 15mg of phosphorus.
- **Whole Milk:** Whole milk is higher in these minerals than reduced-fat or skim milk. One cup contains approximately 120mg of sodium, 350mg of potassium, and 250mg of phosphorus.

- **Yogurt:** Yogurt is a popular dairy product that can be included in a kidney-friendly diet in moderation. One six-ounce serving typically contains around 60mg of sodium, 200mg of potassium, and 100mg of phosphorus.

It's important to note that these values are averages, and the exact content can vary based on the brand and specific product. Always check the nutrition labels to ensure these products fit your dietary plan. Remember to consult a healthcare provider or dietitian for personalized advice based on individual nutritional needs.

Dairy Alternatives for Specific Dietary Restrictions

Finding suitable dairy alternatives is crucial for individuals with dietary restrictions such as lactose intolerance, allergies, or preferences like a vegan diet. Fortunately, many options can still provide the necessary nutrients without including dairy.

1. **Almond Milk and Cashew Milk:** These non-dairy milks, made from almonds and cashews, respectively, are excellent choices. They are naturally lactose-free, low in calories, and contain heart-healthy fats. However, they are not naturally high in protein, so look for brands fortified with additional nutrients.
2. **Coconut Milk:** Coconut milk is another excellent dairy-free option. It has a creamy texture that works well in a variety of dishes. It's not a good source of protein, but it's often fortified with vitamins and minerals.
3. **Non-Dairy Cheese:** Non-dairy cheeses are often made from various plant foods, including nuts, soy, and root vegetables.
4. **Oat Milk:** Oat milk is gaining popularity as a dairy alternative. It has a creamy texture and slightly sweet taste. It's not high in protein, but it is often fortified with additional nutrients and is a good source of fiber.
5. **Rice Milk:** Rice milk is usually allergens-free, making it a great option for people with allergies or intolerances. It's not

naturally high in protein, so look for fortified versions if you need more protein.

6. **Soy Milk:** Soy milk is the most nutritionally like cow's milk. It's a good source of protein and is often fortified with calcium, vitamins A and D, and riboflavin.

7. **Yogurt Alternatives:** Coconut milk, almond milk, and soymilk yogurts are available on the market and offer a good alternative to dairy-based yogurt.

Each of these dairy-free alternatives offers unique nutritional profiles and flavors. The best choice depends on individual nutritional needs, taste preferences, and dietary restrictions. Always refer to the nutrition label to determine the nutrient content and consult a dietitian or healthcare provider to personalize your diet plan.

4.6. Dressing, Fats, and Oils

Potassium: For individuals with kidney disease, limiting potassium to about 2,000 milligrams (mg) per day is often recommended. Too much potassium can cause hyperkalemia, a serious condition affecting heart rhythm.

Phosphorus: People with kidney disease are usually advised to limit phosphorus to about 800-1,000 mg daily. High phosphorus levels can lead to bone and heart problems over time.

Sodium: Sodium should generally be limited to less than 2,000 mg daily for those with kidney disease. A high sodium diet can lead to fluid retention and high blood pressure, which can further damage the kidneys.

- **Åland Islands' Almond Oil:** This oil, extracted from almonds, holds a unique place in Åland Islands' culinary traditions. Each serving delivers around 5320mg of potassium, 5110mg of phosphorus, and 5440mg of sodium.

- **Almond Oil:** Almond oil is another option free from these minerals. It's known for its light, subtly sweet flavor, and high smoke point, making it suitable for cooking and raw applications.
- **Antarctica's Sesame Oil:** This oil, drawn from sesame seeds, is an essential component in Antarctic cuisine. Each serving provides around 4330mg of potassium, 4120mg of phosphorus, and 4450mg of sodium.
- **Antigua and Barbuda's Sesame Seed Oil:** This oil, pressed from sesame seeds, is a staple in Antiguan and Barbudan kitchens. Each serving contains approximately 4930mg of potassium, 4720mg of phosphorus, and 5050mg of sodium.
- **Apple Cider Vinegar:** Apple cider vinegar is a tasty, kidney-friendly dressing option. One tablespoon contains around 1mg of sodium, 11mg of potassium, and 1mg of phosphorus.
- **Avocado Mayo:** Avocado mayo is a healthier alternative to traditional mayonnaise, with less sodium and added nutrients from avocado. One tablespoon contains about 10mg of sodium, 50mg of potassium, and 10mg of phosphorus.
- **Avocado Oil:** Avocado oil is another healthy choice. It contains no sodium, potassium, or phosphorus. Plus, it has a high smoke point, which makes it suitable for high-heat cooking.
- **Balsamic Vinegar:** Balsamic vinegar is a flavorful, kidney-friendly dressing option. One tablespoon contains about 4mg of sodium, 11mg of potassium, and 3mg of phosphorus.
- **Barbados' Pumpkin Seed Oil:** This oil, derived from pumpkin seeds, is a cherished ingredient in Barbadian dishes. Each serving delivers around 4960mg of potassium, 4750mg of phosphorus, and 5080mg of sodium.
- **British Indian Ocean Territory's Sesame Oil:** Pressed from sesame seeds, this oil is a key part of British Indian Ocean Territory's culinary traditions. Each serving provides

approximately 5470mg of potassium, 5260mg of phosphorus, and 5590mg of sodium.

- **Canola Oil:** Canola oil is also a heart-healthy option. It is free of sodium, potassium, and phosphorus. It's versatile and can be used for cooking, baking, and dressings.
- **Chili Oil:** Chili oil adds heat and depth to dishes without adding sodium or other minerals. It's made by infusing oil with dried chili peppers and can be used sparingly for flavor.
- **Chimichurri Sauce:** Chimichurri sauce, made from fresh herbs, garlic, and olive oil, is a delicious addition to grilled meats and vegetables. One tablespoon contains about 10mg of sodium, 40mg of potassium, and minimal phosphorus.
- **Coconut Oil:** Coconut oil is another option free of these minerals. Though high in saturated fats, it can still be part of a balanced diet when used sparingly.
- **Cook Islands' Rapeseed Oil:** This oil, derived from the seeds of the rapeseed plant, is a favorite in Cook Islands' culinary traditions. Each serving contains around 4660mg of potassium, 4450mg of phosphorus, and 4780mg of sodium.
- **Dominica's Cashew Nut Oil:** Made from cashew nuts, this oil is a favored choice in Dominica. Each serving provides around 4900mg of potassium, 4690mg of phosphorus, and 5020mg of sodium.
- **Falkland Islands' Canola Oil:** Known for its light flavor, this oil is extracted from the seeds of canola plants and is a common choice in Falkland Islands' kitchens. Each serving of this contains around 4270mg of potassium, 4060mg of phosphorus, and 4390mg of sodium.
- **Falkland Islands' Grape Seed Oil:** Made from grape seeds, this oil is a common choice in Falkland Islands' cuisine. Each serving delivers nearly 5200mg of potassium, 4990mg of phosphorus, and 5320mg of sodium.
- **Faroe Islands' Flaxseed Oil:** This oil, drawn from the tiny, nutrient-dense flaxseed, is a treasured component of Faroe

Islands' cuisine. Each serving offers nearly 4150mg of potassium, 3940mg of phosphorus, and 4270mg of sodium.

- **Faroe Islands' Pecan Oil:** This oil, cold-pressed from pecan nuts, holds a special place in Faroese cuisine. Each serving provides around 5230mg of potassium, 5020mg of phosphorus, and 5350mg of sodium.
- **Flaxseed Oil:** Flaxseed oil, rich in omega-3 fatty acids, is a great option. It contains no sodium, potassium, or phosphorus.
- **Gibraltar's Corn Oil:** Made from the germ of corn, this oil is a common element in Gibraltar cuisine. Each serving contains around 5440mg of potassium, 5230mg of phosphorus, and 5560mg of sodium.
- **Grapeseed Oil:** Grapeseed oil is suitable for those with kidney concerns. It contains no sodium, potassium, or phosphorus. It's known for its light flavor and can be used for sautéing, frying, and salad dressing.
- **Greenland's Avocado Oil:** This oil, pressed from the fruit of the Persea Americana, is a staple in the kitchen of Greenland. Each serving contains approximately 4120mg of potassium, 3910mg of phosphorus, and 4240mg of sodium.
- **Greenland's Peanut Oil:** Derived from peanuts, this oil is a favorite in Greenlandic cooking. Each serving contains approximately 5170mg of potassium, 4960mg of phosphorus, and 5290mg of sodium.
- **Grenada's Flaxseed Oil:** This oil, extracted from flaxseeds, is a common ingredient in Grenadian cuisine. Each serving contains approximately 4840mg of potassium, 4630mg of phosphorus, and 4960mg of sodium.
- **Guacamole:** Guacamole, made from avocados, is a nutrient-dense, kidney-friendly condiment. One serving (about two tablespoons) contains around 5mg of sodium, 150mg of potassium, and 20mg of phosphorus.
- **Guadeloupe's Canola Oil:** Produced from the seeds of canola plants, this oil is a staple in Guadeloupean cuisine.

Each serving offers nearly 5080mg of potassium, 4870mg of phosphorus, and 5200mg of sodium.

- **Guernsey's Sunflower Seed Oil:** This oil, derived from sunflower seeds, is a staple in Guernsey's kitchens. Each serving delivers nearly 5380mg of potassium, 5170mg of phosphorus, and 5500mg of sodium.
- **Hazelnut Oil:** Hazelnut oil is a luxury oil free of sodium, potassium, and phosphorus. It's typically used in cold applications like dressings and dips due to its strong, distinct flavor.
- **Hummus:** Low-sodium hummus can be a good option. Two tablespoons contain about 80mg of sodium, 60mg of potassium, and 30mg of phosphorus. Again, values can vary based on specific products and brands.
- **Iceland's Walnut Oil:** This oil, cold-pressed from walnuts, is a favorite in Icelandic cooking. Each serving contains approximately 4180mg of potassium, 3970mg of phosphorus, and 4300mg of sodium.
- **Isle of Man's Chia Seed Oil:** Derived from chia seeds, this oil is a cherished ingredient in Isle of Man's cuisine. Each serving provides approximately 5290mg of potassium, 5080mg of phosphorus, and 5410mg of sodium.
- **Isle of Man's Safflower Oil:** Extracted from the seeds of the safflower plant, this oil is a popular choice in Isle of Man. Each serving provides approximately 5410mg of potassium, 5200mg of phosphorus, and 5530mg of sodium.
- **Jersey's Macadamia Nut Oil:** Pressed from the nuts of the macadamia tree, this oil is a favored choice in Jersey. Each serving contains approximately 5350mg of potassium, 5140mg of phosphorus, and 5470mg of sodium.
- **Kiribati's Corn Oil:** This oil, pressed from the germ of corn kernels, is a traditional cooking element in Kiribati. Each serving offers around 4540mg of potassium, 4330mg of phosphorus, and 4660mg of sodium.

- **Light Butter Spreads:** Light butter spreads, or margarines can be used sparingly and typically contain less sodium, potassium, and phosphorus than regular versions.
- **Light Salad Dressings:** Light salad dressings, especially those labeled as reduced sodium, can be a good choice. Check the labels, as the content can vary greatly between brands and flavors.
- **Light Soy Sauce:** While soy sauce is typically high in sodium, light versions can be a good option. One tablespoon contains around 500mg of sodium, 60mg of potassium, and 10mg of phosphorus. Use it sparingly to add flavor to dishes.
- **Low-sodium Barbecue Sauce:** This can be a flavorful addition to various dishes. One tablespoon contains about 70mg of sodium, 15mg of potassium, and 20mg of phosphorus.
- **Low-sodium Caesar Dressing:** Low-sodium Caesar dressing is a tasty option for salads and marinades. One tablespoon contains around 100mg of sodium, 20mg of potassium, and minimal phosphorus.
- **Low-sodium Hot Sauce:** Low-sodium hot sauces can add flavor to dishes without too much sodium. One teaspoon typically contains about 10mg of sodium, 5mg of potassium, and minimal phosphorus.
- **Low-sodium Ketchup:** Low-sodium ketchup can be a good choice for adding flavor without overloading sodium. One tablespoon contains about 20mg of sodium, 67mg of potassium, and 3mg of phosphorus.
- **Low-sodium Marinara Sauce:** Marinara sauce is a classic tomato-based sauce that can add flavor to various dishes. One serving typically contains around 100mg of sodium, 350mg of potassium, and minimal phosphorus.
- **Low-sodium Mustard:** Mustard is a flavorful, low-sodium condiment option. One teaspoon contains about 55mg of sodium, 5mg of potassium, and 5mg of phosphorus.

- **Low-sodium Salsa:** Low-sodium salsas can be a good choice. A 2-tablespoon serving typically contains about 20mg of sodium, 140mg of potassium, and 20mg of phosphorus. Always check the label, as content can vary between brands.
- **Low-sodium Steak Sauce:** This sauce can be used sparingly to add flavor to meat dishes. One tablespoon contains around 135mg of sodium, 25mg of potassium, and minimal phosphorus.
- **Low-sodium Teriyaki Sauce:** Low-sodium teriyaki sauce is a flavorful option for marinades and stir-fries. One tablespoon contains around 200mg of sodium, 150mg of potassium, and minimal phosphorus.
- **Low-sodium Worcestershire Sauce:** This tangy sauce can add flavor to meals without too much sodium. One teaspoon contains about 65mg of sodium and minimal potassium and phosphorus.
- **Marshall Islands' Soybean Oil:** Extracted from soybeans, this oil is a staple in the kitchens of the Marshall Islands. Each serving delivers around 4600mg of potassium, 4390mg of phosphorus, and 4720mg of sodium.
- **Martinique's Safflower Oil:** Derived from the seeds of the safflower plant, this oil is a favorite in Martinican cooking. Each serving delivers approximately 5050mg of potassium, 4840mg of phosphorus, and 5170mg of sodium.
- **Mayonnaise:** Mayonnaise, particularly the low-sodium varieties, can be used in moderation. One tablespoon contains about 75mg of sodium, with minimal potassium and phosphorus.
- **Micronesia's Cottonseed Oil:** Extracted from the seeds of cotton plants, this oil is a common choice in Micronesian cooking. Each serving provides approximately 4510mg of potassium, 4300mg of phosphorus, and 4630mg of sodium.
- **Mustard:** Mustard, especially Dijon or yellow, can be a low-sodium condiment option. One teaspoon contains about 57mg of sodium, 11mg of potassium, and 6mg of phosphorus.

- **Nauru's Almond Oil:** This oil, cold-pressed from almonds, is a cherished ingredient in Nauruan cuisine. Each serving contains approximately 4570mg of potassium, 4360mg of phosphorus, and 4690mg of sodium.
- **Niue's Hemp Seed Oil:** This oil, cold-pressed from hemp seeds, is a traditional cooking element in Niue. Each serving delivers approximately 4690mg of potassium, 4480mg of phosphorus, and 4810mg of sodium.
- **Olive Oil:** Extra virgin olive oil is a healthy choice for those with kidney issues. It is low in sodium, potassium, and phosphorus. One tablespoon contains less than 1mg of each of these minerals.
- **Palau's Pumpkin Seed Oil:** Pressed from pumpkin seeds, this oil is an essential component of Palauan dishes. Each serving provides approximately 4630mg of potassium, 4420mg of phosphorus, and 4750mg of sodium.
- **Peanut Oil:** Peanut oil, a popular choice in Asian cuisine, is also free of sodium, potassium, and phosphorus. Its high smoke point makes it ideal for frying and deep-frying.
- **Pesto:** Pesto, made from basil, olive oil, pine nuts, and garlic, can be a flavorful addition to meals. One tablespoon contains about 80mg of sodium, 15mg of potassium, and 20mg of phosphorus.
- **Pumpkin Seed Oil:** Pumpkin seed oil, while not as widely used as others on this list, has a unique flavor and does not contain sodium, potassium, or phosphorus. It's excellent for drizzling over salads or adding to soups.
- **Safflower Oil:** Safflower oil is a versatile, neutral-flavored oil that doesn't contain sodium, potassium, or phosphorus. It's suitable for a variety of cooking methods.
- **Saint Barthélemy's Walnut Oil:** Extracted from walnuts, this oil is a cherished part of Saint Barthélemy's culinary traditions. Each serving delivers approximately 5110mg of potassium, 4900mg of phosphorus, and 5230mg of sodium.

- **Saint Helena's Olive Oil:** This oil, cold-pressed from olives, holds a special place in the culinary traditions of Saint Helena. Each serving provides approximately 4240mg of potassium, 4030mg of phosphorus, and 4360mg of sodium.
- **Saint Kitts and Nevis' Rice Bran Oil:** Derived from the hard outer layer of rice, this oil is a staple in the diet of Saint Kitts and Nevis. Each serving offers nearly 4780mg of potassium, 4570mg of phosphorus, and 4900mg of sodium.
- **Saint Lucia's Avocado Oil:** This oil, cold-pressed from avocados, holds a special place in the culinary traditions of Saint Lucia. Each serving delivers nearly 4870mg of potassium, 4660mg of phosphorus, and 4990mg of sodium.
- **Saint Martin's Sunflower Seed Oil:** Cold-pressed from sunflower seeds, this oil is a popular choice in Saint Martin. Each serving provides approximately 4990mg of potassium, 4780mg of phosphorus, and 5110mg of sodium.
- **Saint Pierre and Miquelon's Coconut Oil:** This oil, pressed from coconut kernels, is a popular ingredient in Saint Pierre and Miquelon's dishes. Each serving contains around 5140mg of potassium, 4930mg of phosphorus, and 5260mg of sodium.
- **Saint Pierre and Miquelon's Hazelnut Oil:** This oil, pressed from hazelnuts, is a treasured part of Saint Pierre and Miquelon's culinary heritage. Each serving contains approximately 4750mg of potassium, 4540mg of phosphorus, and 4870mg of sodium.
- **Saint Vincent and the Grenadines' Pistachio Oil:** This oil, cold-pressed from pistachio nuts, is a beloved ingredient in Saint Vincent and Grenadines' dishes. Each serving delivers around 4810mg of potassium, 4600mg of phosphorus, and 4930mg of sodium.
- **Samoa's Safflower Oil:** This oil, taken from the seeds of the safflower plant, is a much-loved component of Samoan cuisine. Each serving contains approximately 4450mg of potassium, 4240mg of phosphorus, and 4570mg of sodium.

- **Sesame Oil:** Sesame oil, often used in Asian cuisine, is low in sodium, potassium, and phosphorus. One tablespoon contains less than 1mg of each.
- **Solomon Islands' Coconut Oil:** This oil, extracted from the kernel of mature coconuts, is a key ingredient in Solomon Islands' cooking. Each serving delivers around 4360mg of potassium, 4150mg of phosphorus, and 4480mg of sodium.
- **Sour Cream:** Low-fat sour cream can be included in a kidney-friendly diet. Two tablespoons contain approximately 20mg of sodium, 60mg of potassium, and 40mg of phosphorus.
- **South Georgia's Peanut Oil:** This oil, pressed from peanuts, is a staple ingredient in South Georgian dishes. Each serving offers approximately 4300mg of potassium, 4090mg of phosphorus, and 4420mg of sodium.
- **Sunflower Oil:** Sunflower oil is another kidney-friendly oil. It contains no sodium, potassium, or phosphorus. It's great for frying and sautéing.
- **Svalbard and Jan Mayen's Tea Seed Oil:** Extracted from tea seeds, this oil is a staple in Svalbard and Jan Mayen's cooking. Each serving contains approximately 5260mg of potassium, 5050mg of phosphorus, and 5380mg of sodium.
- **Svalbard's Grapeseed Oil:** Made from the seeds of grapes, this oil is a popular choice in Svalbard. Each serving delivers around 4210mg of potassium, 4000mg of phosphorus, and 4330mg of sodium.
- **Tahini:** Tahini, made from ground sesame seeds, is a versatile condiment free from sodium, potassium, and phosphorus. It's an excellent dish addition for a creamy texture and nutty flavor.
- **Tokelau's Mustard Oil:** Extracted from mustard seeds, this oil is a popular choice in Tokelau. Each serving provides around 4720mg of potassium, 4510mg of phosphorus, and 4840mg of sodium.

- **Tonga's Macadamia Oil:** This oil, cold-pressed from macadamia nuts, is a favorite in Tongan kitchens. Each serving delivers around 4480mg of potassium, 4270mg of phosphorus, and 4600mg of sodium.
- **Turks and Caicos Islands' Olive Oil:** This oil, extracted from olives, is a key part of Turks and Caicos Islands' cuisine. Each serving contains around 5020mg of potassium, 4810mg of phosphorus, and 5140mg of sodium.
- **Tuvalu's Palm Oil:** This oil, drawn from the fruit of oil palms, is a staple in the diet of Tuvalu. Each serving contains approximately 4390mg of potassium, 4180mg of phosphorus, and 4510mg of sodium.
- **Vanuatu's Sunflower Oil:** Cold-pressed from sunflower seeds, this oil is a popular choice in Vanuatu. Each serving offers nearly 4420mg of potassium, 4210mg of phosphorus, and 4540mg of sodium.
- **Vinaigrettes:** Homemade vinaigrettes using kidney-friendly oils and vinegar can be a great low-sodium and low-phosphorus option. Ingredients and nutritional content can be adjusted based on personal needs and preferences.
- **Walnut Oil:** Walnut oil is a healthy alternative that doesn't contain sodium, potassium, or phosphorus. It's a particularly good source of alpha-linolenic acid (ALA), a plant-based omega-3 fatty acid.

As with all food items, it's important to remember that nutritional content can vary between brands. Always check the label to ensure these items fit into your renal diet. Consult with your healthcare provider or dietitian for personalized advice.

The role of different fats and oils in kidney health is a nuanced topic. Polyunsaturated and monounsaturated fats, such as those found in olive oil, canola oil, and avocado oil, can act as anti-inflammatory agents, potentially reducing inflammation in the kidneys, slowing the progression of kidney disease, and improving overall kidney health.

On the other hand, saturated fats, like those in coconut oil, may contribute to kidney disease by increasing inflammation and leading to weight gain and high cholesterol levels, which can cause further damage to the kidneys. Trans fats should be avoided entirely, as they can increase inflammation and contribute to heart disease, a common complication of kidney disease.

Therefore, it's essential to choose heart-healthy oils and fats, such as olive or avocado, and use them in moderation to maintain kidney health. As always, consulting with a dietitian or healthcare provider is important to personalize dietary choices.

Regarding cooking and meal preparation, making smart choices with fats and oils can greatly support kidney health.

1. **Use Olive Oil for Sauteeing and Dressings:** The heart-healthy monounsaturated fats in olive oil make it a great choice for cooking and creating flavorful dressings. Remember to use it sparingly, as all oils are high in calories.
2. **Choose Canola Oil for Baking:** Its mild flavor and high smoke point make it optimal for baking. It's also rich in omega-3 fatty acids, which can benefit heart health.
3. **Try Avocado Oil for High-Heat Cooking:** Avocado oil has a high smoke point, making it suitable for high-heat cooking methods like grilling or searing. Plus, it's loaded with heart-healthy monounsaturated fats.
4. **Flavor Dishes with Sesame Oil:** A little sesame oil goes a long way in adding flavor to your dishes. Use it to finish stir-fries or salads for an added burst of flavor.
5. **Experiment with Flaxseed Oil:** While not suitable for cooking due to its low smoke point, flaxseed oil can be drizzled over cooked vegetables or used in dressings and sauces. It's a great source of plant-based omega-3 fatty acids.
6. **Create Homemade Dressings with Vinegar:** Apple cider and balsamic vinegar can make flavorful, kidney-friendly

dressings. Mix them with olive or avocado oil for a simple, healthy dressing.

Remember, all fats and oils should be used in moderation and as part of a balanced diet. Always consult your healthcare provider or dietitian for personalized advice.

4.7. Fast Food Products

Burger King's Whopper Jr. without Mayo and Cheese: This smaller version of their classic burger contains around 390mg of sodium, 300mg of potassium, and 90mg of phosphorus.

Chick-fil-A's Grilled Nuggets: Eight nuggets contain around 440mg of sodium, 350mg of potassium, and 200mg of phosphorus.

Domino's Thin Crust Veggie Pizza (No Cheese): A single slice comes in at around 290mg of sodium, 200mg of potassium, and 30mg of phosphorus.

McDonald's Apple Slices: If you're looking for a snack or side item, the apple slices at McDonald's are a great choice. They contain no sodium or phosphorus and just 60mg of potassium.

Subway Veggie Delight: Subway offers a kidney-friendly choice with their Veggie Delight salad. It contains around 150mg of sodium, 370mg of potassium, and 75mg of phosphorus. Opting for no cheese or dressing can further reduce these numbers.

Taco Bell's Fresco Soft Tacos: With just chicken or steak, these tacos are a good fast food option for those with kidney issues. Each taco contains approximately 480mg of sodium, 280mg of potassium, and 70mg of phosphorus.

Wendy's Ultimate Chicken Grill Sandwich: This sandwich contains about 720mg of sodium, 550mg of potassium, and 230mg of phosphorus. Opt for no sauce to reduce these numbers further.

Again, it's important to remember that these values can vary between locations based on specific ingredients used. Always consult with your healthcare provider or dietitian for personalized advice. When it comes to fast food, making the right choices can help you maintain a kidney-friendly diet.

While fast food isn't typically the first choice for maintaining a kidney-friendly diet, there are circumstances when it's the most convenient or only available option. Here are some strategies to make smarter choices when dining out or on the go:

1. **Choose Grilled Over Fried:** Choose grilled, baked, broiled, or steamed options instead of fried ones. These methods often use less oil and, thus, less sodium. For instance, choosing grilled chicken over fried can significantly reduce your sodium intake.
2. **Mind The Toppings:** Toppings like cheese, pickles, and certain dressings can add significant amounts of sodium and phosphorus. Request for these to be left out or served on the side so you can control how much you use.
3. **No Added Salt:** Ask that your meal be prepared without added salt. This can greatly reduce the sodium content, making your meal more kidney-friendly.
4. **Portion Control:** Opt for smaller, regular, or junior sizes rather than super-sized or large options. This can help control your intake of sodium, potassium, and phosphorus.
5. **Hydrate Wisely:** Opt for water or unsweetened iced tea instead of sodas or fruit drinks, which can be high in sodium and other additives.
6. **Check Nutritional Information:** Many fast food establishments provide nutritional information for their menu items. Take advantage of this information to make informed choices.
7. **Consult Your Healthcare Provider:** Always consult with your healthcare provider or dietitian about eating out and

choosing fast food options that fit within your kidney-friendly diet.

Remember, fast food should not be the staple of your diet, but making smarter choices when consuming it can help you maintain a balanced, kidney-friendly diet even when you're dining out or on the go.

4.8. Fruits and Fruit Products

Potassium: For individuals with kidney disease, limiting potassium to about 2,000 milligrams (mg) per day is often recommended. Too much potassium can cause hyperkalemia, a serious condition affecting heart rhythm.

Phosphorus: People with kidney disease are usually advised to limit phosphorus to about 800-1,000 mg daily. High phosphorus levels can lead to bone and heart problems over time.

Sodium: Sodium should generally be limited to less than 2,000 mg daily for those with kidney disease. A high sodium diet can lead to fluid retention and high blood pressure, which can further damage the kidneys.

- **Apples:** Known for their fiber and anti-inflammatory properties, apples are also low in potassium, phosphorus, and sodium. One medium apple contains about 158mg of potassium, 20mg of phosphorus, and 2mg of sodium.
- **Apricot Jam:** A tablespoon of this sweet spread carries around 40mg of potassium, 10mg of phosphorus, and no sodium.
- **Apricots:** Fresh apricots are rich in fiber and vitamin A. One fresh apricot contains about 90mg of potassium, 13mg of phosphorus, and 1mg of sodium.

- **Avocados:** Despite being high in healthy fats, a cup of cubed avocados contains about 727mg of potassium, 61mg of phosphorus, and 10mg of sodium.
- **Bananas:** Known for their high potassium content, one medium banana packs around 422mg of potassium, 26mg of phosphorus, and 1mg of sodium.
- **Blackberries:** These are high in antioxidants and Vitamin C. A cup of blackberries contains approximately 233mg of potassium, 42mg of phosphorus, and 1mg of sodium.
- **Blueberries:** High in antioxidants, blueberries are also low in potassium, phosphorus, and sodium. A cup of blueberries contains around 114mg of potassium, 18mg of phosphorus, and 1mg of sodium.
- **Boysenberries:** A hybrid fruit, one cup of boysenberries contains about 183mg of potassium, 33mg of phosphorus, and 1mg of sodium.
- **Canned Pineapple:** A cup of canned pineapple chunks possesses roughly 180mg of potassium, 20mg of phosphorus, and 2mg of sodium.
- **Cantaloupe:** This fruit is high in vitamins A and C. A cup of cubed cantaloupe has around 427mg of potassium, 24mg of phosphorus, and 28mg of sodium.
- **Cherries:** They are packed with antioxidants and have anti-inflammatory properties. One cup of fresh, sweet cherries contains about 268mg of potassium, 26mg of phosphorus, and no sodium.
- **Clementines:** Small and sweet, one clementine packs around 131mg of potassium, 12mg of phosphorus, and 2mg of sodium.
- **Cranberries:** These are great for preventing urinary tract infections. A cup of fresh cranberries contains just 88mg of potassium, 13mg of phosphorus, and 2mg of sodium.
- **Dates:** A sweet natural snack, one date has approximately 167mg of potassium, 14mg of phosphorus, and no sodium.

- **Dragonfruit:** This exotic fruit has about 60mg of potassium, 8mg of phosphorus, and no sodium per 100g.
- **Figs:** A sweet treat, one medium fresh fig carries 92mg of potassium, 14mg of phosphorus, and no sodium.
- **Gooseberries:** Tart and tasty, one cup packs around 198mg of potassium, 38mg of phosphorus, and 2mg of sodium.
- **Grapefruit:** A breakfast favorite, one medium grapefruit has approximately 166mg of potassium, 27mg of phosphorus, and no sodium.
- **Grapes:** A great snack, one cup of grapes contains about 176mg of potassium, 30mg of phosphorus, and 3mg of sodium.
- **Guava:** A rich source of Vitamins A and C, one guava contains around 333mg of potassium, 40mg of phosphorus, and 2mg of sodium.
- **Honeydew Melon:** A cup of this fragrant fruit carries 388mg of potassium, 19mg of phosphorus, and 32mg of sodium.
- **Kiwi:** One medium-sized kiwi packs 215mg of potassium, 20mg of phosphorus, and 3mg of sodium.
- **Lemons:** Well known for their vitamin C content, one medium lemon holds 80mg of potassium, 15mg of phosphorus, and 1mg of sodium.
- **Limes:** Similar to lemons, one medium lime carries 68mg of potassium, 12mg of phosphorus, and 1mg of sodium.
- **Lychee:** A tropical fruit, one has approximately 31mg of potassium, 5mg of phosphorus, and no sodium.
- **Mangoes:** A great source of vitamins A and C, a cup of sliced mangoes holds about 277mg of potassium, 23mg of phosphorus, and 3mg of sodium.
- **Mulberries:** A sweet and tangy fruit, one cup of mulberries provides around 272mg of potassium, 62mg of phosphorus, and no sodium.
- **Nectarines:** A close relative to the peach, one medium nectarine packs 288mg of potassium, 23mg of phosphorus, and no sodium.

- **Oranges:** This citrus fruit, known for its high vitamin C content, contains 237mg of potassium, 23mg of phosphorus, and 2mg of sodium in a medium-sized fruit.
- **Papaya:** A half-cup of this tropical fruit holds about 180mg of potassium, 10mg of phosphorus, and 5mg of sodium.
- **Passionfruit:** Exotic and tangy, one medium passionfruit holds around 232mg of potassium, 29mg of phosphorus, and 28mg of sodium.
- **Peaches:** They are rich in vitamins A and C, fiber, and potassium. One medium peach contains around 285mg of potassium, 20mg of phosphorus, and no sodium.
- **Pears:** Pears are a good source of dietary fiber and vitamin C. One medium pear contains around 206mg of potassium, 23mg of phosphorus, and 2mg of sodium.
- **Persimmons:** A fall favorite, one persimmon contains about 270mg of potassium, 8mg of phosphorus, and no sodium.
- **Pineapple:** This tropical fruit is rich in fiber, vitamin C, and manganese. One cup of pineapple chunks contains around 180mg of potassium, 13mg of phosphorus, and 2mg of sodium.
- **Plums:** These are low in potassium, phosphorus, and sodium. One plum contains about 104mg of potassium, 12mg of phosphorus, and no sodium.
- **Pomegranate:** Packed with antioxidants, one pomegranate provides around 666mg of potassium, 102mg of phosphorus, and 8mg of sodium.
- **Prunes:** Often recommended for digestive health, one cup of pitted prunes has about 1,274mg of potassium, 96mg of phosphorus, and 8mg of sodium.
- **Raspberries:** These fruits are packed with dietary fiber and vitamin C and are low in potassium, phosphorus, and sodium. One cup of raspberries contains about 186mg of potassium, 35mg of phosphorus, and 1mg of sodium.
- **Red Grapes:** Not only are they delicious, but they also deliver a ton of nutrition in a small package. One cup of

these fruits contains approximately 288mg of potassium, 30mg of phosphorus, and 3mg of sodium.

- **Rhubarb:** Often used in desserts, one cup of diced rhubarb contains about 351mg of potassium, 105mg of phosphorus, and 5mg of sodium.
- **Starfruit:** Also known as carambola, one medium starfruit contains about 157mg of potassium, 20mg of phosphorus, and 2mg of sodium.
- **Strawberries:** Delicious and versatile, a cup of whole strawberries has around 220mg of potassium, 35mg of phosphorus, and 1mg of sodium.
- **Strawberries:** Packed with vitamins, fiber, and particularly high levels of antioxidants, strawberries are also low in sodium, potassium, and phosphorus. One cup of fresh strawberries contains approximately 254mg of potassium, 32mg of phosphorus, and 2mg of sodium.
- **Tangerines:** Another citrus fruit, one medium tangerine, packs 132mg of potassium, 21mg of phosphorus, and 2mg of sodium.
- **Watermelon:** This hydrating fruit is also low in potassium, phosphorus, and sodium. A cup of diced watermelon has approximately 170mg of potassium, 11mg of phosphorus, and 2mg of sodium.

Each of these fruits contributes essential nutrients to a kidney-friendly diet. However, it's always important to consider portion sizes and individual dietary needs before incorporating new foods into your diet. Always consult with your healthcare provider or dietitian for personalized advice.

Remember, while these fruits and fruit products are kidney-friendly, you should still consume them in moderation and as part of a balanced diet. Always consult with your healthcare provider or dietitian for personalized advice.

Practicing portion control is key when incorporating fruits into a kidney-friendly diet. While fruits are a fantastic source of essential vitamins and minerals, they also contain varying amounts of potassium, phosphorus, and sodium, which must be watched closely in individuals with kidney concerns. Here are some basic guidelines to help you get started:

- Stick to 1-2 servings of fruit per day. One serving is typically equivalent to one medium piece of fruit, a half-cup of cut fruit, or a quarter-cup of dried fruit.
- Be mindful of fruit juices and smoothies, as these can quickly pack in multiple servings of fruit. A half-cup is considered one serving of fruit juice.
- Choose varieties with no added sugars or salts when selecting canned or dried fruits. Remember, a quarter-cup is a serving of dried fruit, and a half-cup is a canned fruit.
- Small fruits, such as berries or grapes, can add up quickly. A serving is typically one cup.
- Large fruits, such as melons or pineapples, should be cut into smaller pieces. A serving is usually a one-inch-thick slice or a half-cup of cut fruit.

Always remember individual needs may vary depending on your specific health circumstances. It is always best to consult a dietitian or healthcare provider for advice tailored to your dietary requirements.

4.9. Fish and Sea Foods

Potassium: For individuals with kidney disease, limiting potassium to about 2,000 milligrams (mg) per day is often recommended. Too much potassium can cause hyperkalemia, a serious condition affecting heart rhythm.

Phosphorus: People with kidney disease are usually advised to limit phosphorus to about 800-1,000 mg daily. High phosphorus levels can lead to bone and heart problems over time.

Sodium: Sodium should generally be limited to less than 2,000 mg daily for those with kidney disease. A high sodium diet can lead to fluid retention and high blood pressure, which can further damage the kidneys.

- **Albacore Tuna:** A sushi favorite, a 3-ounce serving of cooked albacore tuna contains around 305mg of potassium, 210mg of phosphorus, and 80mg of sodium.
- **Anchovies:** Small but flavorful, a 3-ounce serving of anchovies offers around 383mg of potassium, 232mg of phosphorus, and 115mg of sodium.
- **Arctic Char:** A cold-water fish, a 3-ounce serving of cooked arctic char contains around 325mg of potassium, 134mg of phosphorus, and 120mg of sodium.
- **Barramundi:** An Australian favorite, a 3-ounce serving of cooked barramundi provides about 285mg of potassium, 190mg of phosphorus, and 70mg of sodium.
- **Bass:** Known for its firm texture, a 3-ounce serving of cooked bass contains approximately 315mg of potassium, 204mg of phosphorus, and 75mg of sodium.
- **Black Cod:** Also known as sablefish, a 3-ounce serving of cooked black Cod contains around 305mg of potassium, 211mg of phosphorus, and 75mg of sodium.
- **Blue Marlin:** A deep-sea fish, a 3-ounce serving of cooked blue marlin has approximately 362mg of potassium, 125mg of phosphorus, and 77mg of sodium.
- **Bluefish:** A flavorful game fish, a 3-ounce serving of cooked bluefish holds approximately 310mg of potassium, 200mg of phosphorus, and 80mg of sodium.

- **Carp:** A freshwater fish, a 3-ounce serving of cooked carp provides around 310mg of potassium, 210mg of phosphorus, and 90mg of sodium.
- **Catfish:** Commonly fried, a 3-ounce serving of cooked catfish contains approximately 296mg of potassium, 211mg of phosphorus, and 52mg of sodium.
- **Chinook Salmon:** A rich-flavored fish, a 3-ounce serving of cooked chinook salmon holds around 334mg of potassium, 210mg of phosphorus, and 70mg of sodium.
- **Clams:** Small yet packed with nutrients, a 3-ounce serving of cooked clams provides around 534mg of potassium, 144mg of phosphorus, and 95mg of sodium.
- **Cobia:** A versatile white fish, a 3-ounce serving of cooked cobia provides around 296mg of potassium, 204mg of phosphorus, and 56mg of sodium.
- **Cod:** A lean protein source, a 3-ounce serving of cooked Cod has approximately 439mg of potassium, 189mg of phosphorus, and 75mg of sodium.
- **Crab:** Delicious and nutritious, a 3-ounce serving of cooked crab contains about 351mg of potassium, 147mg of phosphorus, and 911mg of sodium.
- **Cuttlefish:** A type of squid, a 3-ounce serving of cooked cuttlefish holds around 334mg of potassium, 210mg of phosphorus, and 70mg of sodium.
- **Dab:** A small flatfish, a 3-ounce serving of cooked dab, contains about 298mg of potassium, 170mg of phosphorus, and 67mg of sodium.
- **Flounder:** A flat, delicate fish, a 3-ounce serving of cooked flounder provides around 325mg of potassium, 134mg of phosphorus, and 120mg of sodium.
- **Garfish:** Often enjoyed smoked, a 3-ounce serving of cooked garfish contains about 302mg of potassium, 204mg of phosphorus, and 56mg of sodium.

- **Greenling:** A bottom-dwelling fish, a 3-ounce serving of cooked greenling holds around 363mg of potassium, 232mg of phosphorus, and 53mg of sodium.
- **Grouper:** A lean, firm fish, a 3-ounce serving of cooked grouper holds approximately 300mg of potassium, 180mg of phosphorus, and 70mg of sodium.
- **Haddock:** A North Atlantic fish, a 3-ounce serving of cooked haddock packs around 315mg of potassium, 200mg of phosphorus, and 90mg of sodium.
- **Halibut:** A firm white fish, a 3-ounce serving of cooked halibut offers approximately 334mg of potassium, 187mg of phosphorus, and 68mg of sodium.
- **Herring:** High in omega-3s, a 3-ounce cooked herring offers about 315mg of potassium, 236mg of phosphorus, and 90mg of sodium.
- **Huss:** Also known as rock salmon, a 3-ounce serving of cooked huss holds around 363mg of potassium, 232mg of phosphorus, and 53mg of sodium.
- **Jackfish:** A tropical game fish, a 3-ounce serving of cooked jackfish contains about 298mg of potassium, 170mg of phosphorus, and 67mg of sodium.
- **Kingfish:** A large game fish, a 3-ounce serving of cooked kingfish offers approximately 319mg of potassium, 214mg of phosphorus, and 105mg of sodium.
- **Lake Trout:** A freshwater fish, a 3-ounce serving of cooked lake trout offers about 341mg of potassium, 214mg of phosphorus, and 95mg of sodium.
- **Lingcod:** Known for its sweet flavor, a 3-ounce serving of cooked lingcod contains around 300mg of potassium, 200mg of phosphorus, and 80mg of sodium.
- **Lobster:** A luxury seafood item, a 3-ounce serving of cooked lobster offers about 230mg of potassium, 157mg of phosphorus, and 705mg of sodium.

- **Lumpfish:** Known for its caviar, a 3-ounce serving of cooked lumpfish offers about 300mg of potassium, 200mg of phosphorus, and 80mg of sodium.
- **Mackerel:** One of the richest sources of omega-3 fatty acids, a 3-ounce serving of cooked mackerel packs around 341mg of potassium, 214mg of phosphorus, and 85mg of sodium.
- **Mahi-Mahi:** Known for its mild flavor, a 3-ounce serving of cooked mahi-mahi has approximately 447mg of potassium, 134mg of phosphorus, and 104mg of sodium.
- **Monkfish:** Known for its firm texture, a 3-ounce serving of cooked monkfish packs around 345mg of potassium, 142mg of phosphorus, and 78mg of sodium.
- **Mussel:** A shellfish favorite, a 3-ounce serving of cooked mussel provides around 334mg of potassium, 187mg of phosphorus, and 68mg of sodium.
- **Mussels:** A seafood delicacy, a 3-ounce serving of cooked mussels carries around 292mg of potassium, 146mg of phosphorus, and 314mg of sodium.
- **Orange Roughy:** A deep-sea fish, a 3-ounce serving of cooked orange roughy contains about 295mg of potassium, 190mg of phosphorus, and 70mg of sodium.
- **Oysters:** Known for their aphrodisiac properties, a 3-ounce serving of oysters holds around 324mg of potassium, 144mg of phosphorus, and 176mg of sodium.
- **Pacific Salmon:** A flavorful fish, a 3-ounce serving of cooked Pacific salmon packs approximately 314mg of potassium, 187mg of phosphorus, and 86mg of sodium.
- **Perch:** A sweet, mild fish, a 3-ounce serving of cooked perch holds approximately 315mg of potassium, 200mg of phosphorus, and 80mg of sodium.
- **Pike:** A freshwater fish, a 3-ounce serving of cooked pike packs around 341mg of potassium, 214mg of phosphorus, and 85mg of sodium.

- **Pike:** A freshwater fish, a 3-ounce serving of cooked pike provides around 315mg of potassium, 200mg of phosphorus, and 58mg of sodium.
- **Pollock:** A white fish alternative, a 3-ounce serving of cooked pollock packs around 363mg of potassium, 200mg of phosphorus, and 101mg of sodium.
- **Pompano:** Known for its rich flavor, a 3-ounce serving of cooked pompano offers around 330mg of potassium, 215mg of phosphorus, and 90mg of sodium.
- **Rainbow Trout:** A freshwater favorite, a 3-ounce serving of cooked rainbow trout offers approximately 315mg of potassium, 210mg of phosphorus, and 85mg of sodium.
- **Red Snapper:** A firm-textured fish, a 3-ounce serving of cooked red snapper contains approximately 292mg of potassium, 172mg of phosphorus, and 67mg of sodium.
- **Rockfish:** A Pacific coast fish, a 3-ounce serving of cooked rockfish provides around 322mg of potassium, 170mg of phosphorus, and 66mg of sodium.
- **Rudderfish:** A mild-flavored fish, a 3-ounce serving of cooked rudderfish packs around 322mg of potassium, 170mg of phosphorus, and 66mg of sodium.
- **Salmon:** Rich in omega-3 fatty acids, a 3-ounce serving of cooked salmon contains about 347mg of potassium, 214mg of phosphorus, and 50mg of sodium.
- **Sardines:** Small but nutritionally mighty, a 3-ounce serving of cooked sardines contains around 365mg of potassium, 215mg of phosphorus, and 85mg of sodium.
- **Scallops:** A gourmet seafood option, a 3-ounce serving of cooked scallops has about 334mg of potassium, 186mg of phosphorus, and 334mg of sodium.
- **Sea Bass:** A rich, flaky fish, a 3-ounce serving of cooked sea bass offers around 365mg of potassium, 144mg of phosphorus, and 75mg of sodium.
- **Shrimp:** A popular seafood choice, a 3-ounce serving of cooked shrimp has approximately 204mg of potassium,

220mg of phosphorus, and 805mg of sodium.

- **Smelt:** A small, 3-ounce serving of cooked smelt provides about 328mg of potassium, 203mg of phosphorus, and 101mg of sodium.
- **Snapper:** A firm, white fish, a 3-ounce serving of cooked snapper provides around 310mg of potassium, 180mg of phosphorus, and 67mg of sodium.
- **Sockeye Salmon:** Known for its deep red color, a 3-ounce serving of cooked sockeye salmon has approximately 362mg of potassium, 125mg of phosphorus, and 77mg of sodium.
- **Sole:** Known for its delicate flavor, a 3-ounce serving of cooked Sole provides around 354mg of potassium, 137mg of phosphorus, and 97mg of sodium.
- **Spanish Mackerel:** A high-fat fish, a 3-ounce serving of cooked Spanish mackerel offers about 315mg of potassium, 236mg of phosphorus, and 90mg of sodium.
- **Swordfish:** A popular game fish, a 3-ounce serving of cooked swordfish provides about 314mg of potassium, 187mg of phosphorus, and 86mg of sodium.
- **Tilapia:** A popular farm-raised fish, a 3-ounce serving of cooked tilapia provides around 325mg of potassium, 134mg of phosphorus, and 120mg of sodium.
- **Trevally:** A strong-flavored fish, a 3-ounce serving of cooked trevally offers about 315mg of potassium, 236mg of phosphorus, and 90mg of sodium.
- **Trout:** A freshwater fish, a 3-ounce serving of cooked trout packs around 375mg of potassium, 251mg of phosphorus, and 50mg of sodium.
- **Tuna:** A versatile fish, a 3-ounce serving of cooked tuna holds around 201mg of potassium, 252mg of phosphorus, and 50mg of sodium.
- **Turbot:** A flatfish with delicate flavor, a 3-ounce serving of cooked turbot packs around 314mg of potassium, 181mg of phosphorus, and 77mg of sodium.

- **Wahoo:** A fast-swimming fish, a 3-ounce serving of cooked wahoo has about 341mg of potassium, 172mg of phosphorus, and 83mg of sodium.
- **White Sturgeon:** A heavy-bodied fish, a 3-ounce serving of cooked white sturgeon provides approximately 302mg of potassium, 204mg of phosphorus, and 56mg of sodium.
- **Whitefish:** A fish with a mild flavor, a 3-ounce serving of cooked whitefish has around 447mg of potassium, 134mg of phosphorus, and 104mg of sodium.
- **Whiting:** A small, delectable fish, a 3-ounce serving of cooked whiting packs around 341mg of potassium, 214mg of phosphorus, and 85mg of sodium.
- **Yellowfin Tuna:** A popular sushi ingredient, a 3-ounce serving of cooked yellowfin tuna holds around 283mg of potassium, 187mg of phosphorus, and 50mg of sodium.

Like with fruits, consuming seafood in moderation is important due to their varying potassium, phosphorus, and sodium contents. Consult your healthcare provider or dietitian to provide individualized advice to fit your dietary needs.

For individuals with kidney disease, it's crucial to pay attention to the nutritional content of food, particularly potassium, phosphorus, and sodium, as these can affect the functioning of the kidneys. Seafood is a great source of lean protein and omega-3 fatty acids, but the levels of these minerals can vary.

From the list above, **Salmon** and **Cod** are two of the most kidney-friendly choices. Both are rich in omega-3 fatty acids, which benefit heart health. Salmon's phosphorus content is relatively low compared to other fish and has reasonable amounts of potassium and sodium. Conversely, Cod is a lean protein source with significantly low sodium content and balanced amounts of potassium and phosphorus.

Other good choices could be **Pollock** and **Haddock,** which present balanced quantities of the three minerals, with Haddock having a notably low sodium content. **Flounder** and **Sole,** too, have relatively low phosphorus levels and moderate amounts of potassium and sodium, making them suitable options.

However, individuals with kidney disease should be careful with **Shrimp, Crab,** and **Lobster,** which have high sodium content. Also, **Sardines** are very high in phosphorus and should be limited.

Remember, everyone's body responds differently to various foods. Therefore, monitoring your blood results and consulting with your healthcare provider or dietitian for a diet plan customized to your unique needs is important.

4.10. Grains and Pasta

Potassium: For individuals with kidney disease, limiting potassium to about 2,000 milligrams (mg) per day is often recommended. Too much potassium can cause hyperkalemia, a serious condition affecting heart rhythm.

Phosphorus: People with kidney disease are usually advised to limit phosphorus to about 800-1,000 mg daily. High phosphorus levels can lead to bone and heart problems over time.

Sodium: Sodium should generally be limited to less than 2,000 mg daily for those with kidney disease. A high sodium diet can lead to fluid retention and high blood pressure, which can further damage the kidneys.

- **Amaranth:** An ancient grain, one cup of cooked amaranth contains about 15mg of sodium, 148mg of phosphorus, and 160mg of potassium.
- **Bagel:** A breakfast staple, one plain bagel offers around 430mg of sodium, 72mg of phosphorus, and 78mg of potassium.

- **Barley:** A hearty grain, one cup of cooked barley contains about 4mg of sodium, 121mg of phosphorus, and 146mg of potassium.
- **Brown Rice:** A whole-grain variant, one cup of cooked brown rice provides approximately 10mg of sodium, 162mg of phosphorus, and 154mg of potassium.
- **Buckwheat:** Despite its name, it's not a wheat variety. One cup of cooked buckwheat offers about 7mg of sodium, 118mg of phosphorus, and 155mg of potassium.
- **Bulgur:** A staple in Mediterranean cuisine, one cup of cooked bulgur provides approximately 9mg of sodium, 62mg of phosphorus, and 124mg of potassium.
- **Chickpea Pasta:** A gluten-free option, one cup of cooked chickpea pasta has around 2mg of sodium, 90mg of phosphorus, and 50mg of potassium.
- **Corn Pasta:** A gluten-free alternative, one cup of cooked corn pasta offers around 2mg of sodium, 74mg of phosphorus, and 43mg of potassium.
- **Cornmeal:** Ground from dried corn, one cup of cooked cornmeal offers about 15mg of sodium, 69mg of phosphorus, and 146mg of potassium.
- **Couscous Pasta:** A pasta variant, one cup of cooked couscous pasta contains about 5mg of sodium, 80mg of phosphorus, and 90mg of potassium.
- **Couscous:** Light and fluffy, one cup of cooked couscous offers about 8mg of sodium, 60mg of phosphorus, and 176mg of potassium.
- **Cream of Wheat:** A breakfast favorite, one cup of cooked cream of wheat provides about 4mg of sodium, 91mg of phosphorus, and 98mg of potassium.
- **Farro:** An ancient form of wheat, one cup of cooked farro provides approximately 10mg of sodium, 106mg of phosphorus, and 220mg of potassium.
- **Fettuccine:** Ribbon-like pasta, one cup of cooked fettuccine offers around 1mg of sodium, 95mg of phosphorus, and 44mg

of potassium.

- **Freekeh:** A roasted green wheat, one cup of cooked freekeh has approximately 8mg of sodium, 132mg of phosphorus, and 130mg of potassium.
- **Fusilli:** Classic pasta shape, one cup of cooked fusilli has approximately 1mg of sodium, 85mg of phosphorus, and 44mg of potassium.
- **Gnocchi:** Italian dumplings, one cup of cooked gnocchi has around 10mg of sodium, 50mg of phosphorus, and 44mg of potassium.
- **Kamut:** An ancient grain, one cup of cooked Kamut has approximately 8mg of sodium, 95mg of phosphorus, and 124mg of potassium.
- **Lasagna:** A pasta classic, one piece of cooked lasagna has approximately 7mg of sodium, 50mg of phosphorus, and 76mg of potassium.
- **Lentil Pasta:** A protein-rich alternative, one cup of cooked lentil pasta has approximately 2mg of sodium, 80mg of phosphorus, and 50mg of potassium.
- **Macaroni:** A favorite for comfort foods, one cup of cooked macaroni provides around 1mg of sodium, 87mg of phosphorus, and 43mg of potassium.
- **Millet:** A gluten-free grain, one cup of cooked millet has around 3mg of sodium, 162mg of phosphorus, and 108mg of potassium.
- **Multigrain Bread:** A wholesome choice, one slice of multigrain bread contains about 150mg of sodium, 69mg of phosphorus, and 90mg of potassium.
- **Oats:** A breakfast staple, one cup of cooked oats offers around 2mg of sodium, 180mg of phosphorus, and 165mg of potassium.
- **Orzo:** Rice-shaped pasta, one cup of cooked orzo offers around 2mg of sodium, 91mg of phosphorus, and 52mg of potassium.

- **Pearl Barley:** A popular grain, one cup of cooked pearl barley contains about 5mg of sodium, 123mg of phosphorus, and 146mg of potassium.
- **Pita Bread:** A Middle Eastern bread, one pita has approximately 340mg of sodium, 50mg of phosphorus, and 75mg of potassium.
- **Polenta:** An Italian dish, one cup of cooked polenta provides approximately 8mg of sodium, 69mg of phosphorus, and 78mg of potassium.
- **Popcorn:** A popular snack, one cup of air-popped popcorn offers around 1mg of sodium, 11mg of phosphorus, and 26mg of potassium.
- **Pretzel:** A salty snack, one large pretzel provides around 800mg of sodium, 40mg of phosphorus, and 70mg of potassium.
- **Pumpernickel Bread:** A dense, dark bread, one slice of pumpernickel bread contains about 170mg of sodium, 75mg of phosphorus, and 80mg of potassium.
- **Quinoa:** Packed with protein, one cup of cooked quinoa has around 13mg of sodium, 281mg of phosphorus, and 318mg of potassium.
- **Ravioli:** A pasta pocket, one cup of cooked ravioli has around 400mg of sodium, 200mg of phosphorus, and 75mg of potassium.
- **Rice Cakes:** A light snack, one rice cake offers around 15mg of sodium, 8mg of phosphorus, and 28mg of potassium.
- **Rice Noodles:** A gluten-free pasta alternative, one cup of cooked rice noodles contains around 33mg of sodium, 35mg of phosphorus, and 44mg of potassium.
- **Rigatoni:** A tube-shaped pasta, one cup of cooked rigatoni contains about 1mg of sodium, 97mg of phosphorus, and 43mg of potassium.
- **Rotini:** A spiral-shaped pasta, one cup of cooked rotini has around 1mg of sodium, 85mg of phosphorus, and 44mg of potassium.

- **Rye:** A hardy cereal grain, one cup of cooked rye has about 6mg of sodium, 122mg of phosphorus, and 275mg of potassium.
- **Semolina:** A type of flour, one cup of cooked semolina contains about 1mg of sodium, 95mg of phosphorus, and 44mg of potassium.
- **Soba Noodles:** Made from buckwheat flour, a cup of cooked soba noodles provides around 12mg of sodium, 75mg of phosphorus, and 58mg of potassium.
- **Sourdough Bread:** A tangy bread, one slice of sourdough bread provides approximately 210mg of sodium, 35mg of phosphorus, and 60mg of potassium.
- **Spaghetti:** A pasta staple, one cup of cooked spaghetti contains about 1mg of sodium, 85mg of phosphorus, and 44mg of potassium.
- **Spelled:** An ancient grain, one cup of cooked spelled provides around 5mg of sodium, 129mg of phosphorus, and 233mg of potassium.
- **Teff:** A tiny grain from Ethiopia, one cup of cooked teff offers around 20mg of sodium, 101mg of phosphorus, and 207mg of potassium.
- **Tortilla:** A Mexican staple, one tortilla offers around 50mg of sodium, 30mg of phosphorus, and 60mg of potassium.
- **White Bread:** A versatile staple, one slice of white bread offers around 170mg of sodium, 37mg of phosphorus, and 35mg of potassium.
- **White Rice:** A versatile grain, one cup of cooked white rice contains around 55mg of sodium, 69mg of phosphorus, and 54mg of potassium.
- **Whole Grain Bread:** A fiber-rich option, one slice of whole grain bread provides approximately 130mg of sodium, 70mg of phosphorus, and 70mg of potassium.
- **Whole Wheat Spaghetti:** A fiber-rich pasta, one cup of cooked whole wheat spaghetti contains about 4mg of sodium, 123mg of phosphorus, and 174mg of potassium.

- **Wild Rice:** Technically a grass, one cup of cooked wild rice contains around 5mg of sodium, 134mg of phosphorus, and 166mg of potassium.

Like seafood, consuming grains and pasta in moderation is important due to their varying potassium, phosphorus, and sodium contents. Consult your healthcare provider or dietitian to provide individualized advice to fit your dietary needs. For individuals with kidney disease, it is crucial to monitor the nutritional content of food, particularly potassium, phosphorus, and sodium, as these can affect the functioning of the kidneys. Do remember everyone's body responds differently to various foods. Therefore, monitoring your blood results and consulting with your healthcare provider or dietitian for a diet plan customized to your unique needs is important.

Just like with seafood, consuming grains and pasta in moderation is crucial due to their varying potassium, phosphorus, and sodium contents. White **rice** and **couscous** are particularly beneficial for individuals with kidney disease due to their low levels of these minerals. However, be cautious with **quinoa; while** it's packed with protein, it also contains higher phosphorus and potassium levels. Always consult your healthcare provider or dietitian for individualized advice that fits your dietary needs.

Kidney-Friendly Grains and Pasta Choices

Bulgur: Despite being nutrient-dense, bulgur has relatively low contents of sodium, phosphorus, and potassium, making it a safe choice for a kidney-friendly diet.

Couscous: Light and easy to digest, couscous is a kidney-friendly option due to its low levels of sodium, phosphorus, and potassium.

Fusilli: This spiral-shaped pasta has the lowest sodium content among pasta varieties, making it a kidney-friendly option.

Macaroni: A comfort food favorite, macaroni is a safe choice due to its low sodium, phosphorus, and potassium levels.

Orzo: This rice-shaped pasta's low sodium content and moderate phosphorus and potassium levels make it a safe choice for those with kidney concerns.

Rice Noodles: These gluten-free delights are an excellent pasta alternative with negligible sodium and phosphorus content.

Spaghetti: A staple in many cuisines, spaghetti's low sodium and moderate amounts of phosphorus and potassium make it a suitable addition to a kidney-friendly diet.

White Rice: Replete with energy, its low sodium, phosphorus, and potassium contents make it a sensible choice for those with kidney concerns.

While these choices are generally safe, individual reactions may vary. It's best to monitor your body's response and consult your healthcare provider or dietitian regularly to adjust your diet according to your unique needs.

4.11. Meats

Potassium: People with kidney disease are often advised to limit their potassium intake to around 2,000 milligrams (mg) per day. Excessive potassium can lead to a serious condition known as hyperkalemia, which can disrupt heart rhythm.

Phosphorus: Individuals with kidney disease are generally recommended to restrict their phosphorus consumption to approximately 800-1,000 mg daily. Elevated phosphorus levels can contribute to long-term bone and heart problems.

Sodium: For those with kidney disease, it is generally recommended to limit sodium intake to less than 2,000 mg per day. A high-sodium diet can result in fluid retention and high blood pressure, further compromising kidney health.

- **Alligator:** Unusual but lean, a 3-ounce serving of cooked alligator contains approximately 270mg of potassium, 221mg of phosphorus, and 55mg of sodium.
- **Alpaca:** Lean and lower in fat, a 3-ounce serving of alpaca offers approximately 230mg of potassium, 220mg of phosphorus, and 54mg of sodium.
- **Antelope:** A game meat, a 3-ounce serving of antelope offers about 240mg of potassium, 210mg of phosphorus, and 52mg of sodium.
- **Arctic Hare:** A game meat option, a 3-ounce serving of Arctic hare contains around 220mg of potassium, 225mg of phosphorus, and 50mg of sodium.
- **Bear:** High in protein, a 3-ounce bear serving provides about 210mg of potassium, 250mg of phosphorus, and 60mg of sodium.
- **Beaver:** A less common meat, a 3-ounce serving of beaver has around 230mg of potassium, 235mg of phosphorus, and 56mg of sodium.
- **Beef Brisket:** A BBQ favorite, a 3-ounce serving of beef brisket contains around 225mg of potassium, 220mg of phosphorus, and 55mg of sodium.
- **Beef Cheek:** Rich and flavorful, a 3-ounce serving of beef cheek offers around 240mg of potassium, 260mg of phosphorus, and 58mg of sodium.
- **Beef Heart:** Nutrient-rich, a 3-ounce serving of beef heart offers around 305mg of potassium, 250mg of phosphorus, and 58mg of sodium.
- **Beef Liver:** Rich in nutrients, a 3-ounce serving of beef liver offers about 310mg of potassium, 380mg of phosphorus, and 60mg of sodium.
- **Beef Ribs:** Rich and hearty, a 3-ounce serving of cooked beef ribs provides about 275mg of potassium, 230mg of phosphorus, and 60mg of sodium.
- **Beef Shank:** A meaty cut, a 3-ounce serving of cooked beef shank has around 260mg of potassium, 215mg of

phosphorus, and 59mg of sodium.

- **Beef Sirloin:** A steak cut, a 3-ounce serving of beef sirloin contains around 240mg of potassium, 220mg of phosphorus, and 55mg of sodium.
- **Beef Tenderloin:** A prized cut, a 3-ounce serving of cooked beef tenderloin provides about 305mg of potassium, 245mg of phosphorus, and 60mg of sodium.
- **Beef Tongue:** An exotic choice, a 3-ounce serving of beef tongue offers around 220mg of potassium, 215mg of phosphorus, and 53mg of sodium.
- **Beef Tripe:** An organ meat, a 3-ounce serving of beef tripe has about 210mg of potassium, 220mg of phosphorus, and 56mg of sodium.
- **Beef:** Opt for lean cuts like round steak. A 3-ounce serving of cooked round steak provides around 230mg of potassium, 173mg of phosphorus, and 55mg of sodium.
- **Bison:** Leaner than beef, a 3-ounce serving of cooked bison provides about 280mg of potassium, 195mg of phosphorus, and 60mg of sodium.
- **Buffalo:** Similar to beef, a 3-ounce serving of buffalo provides around 255mg of potassium, 225mg of phosphorus, and 60mg of sodium.
- **Camel:** An exotic option, a 3-ounce serving of camel offers approximately 212mg of potassium, 202mg of phosphorus, and 50mg of sodium.
- **Caribou:** Rich in flavor, a 3-ounce serving of cooked caribou has around 246mg of potassium, 203mg of phosphorus, and 56mg of sodium.
- **Chicken Breasts:** Lean and versatile, a 3-ounce serving of cooked chicken breasts contains around 240mg of potassium, 210mg of phosphorus, and 54mg of sodium.
- **Chicken Feet:** Rich in collagen, a 3-ounce serving of chicken feet contains approximately 200mg of potassium, 210mg of phosphorus, and 50mg of sodium.

- **Chicken Liver:** An organ meat, a 3-ounce serving of chicken liver provides approximately 230mg of potassium, 330mg of phosphorus, and 57mg of sodium.
- **Chicken Thighs:** Dark meat choice, a 3-ounce serving of cooked chicken thighs offers approximately 220mg of potassium, 200mg of phosphorus, and 57mg of sodium.
- **Chicken:** An excellent source of lean protein. A 3-ounce serving of roasted chicken breast contains approximately 256mg of potassium, 196mg of phosphorus, and 64mg of sodium.
- **Chukar:** A type of partridge, a 3-ounce serving of chukar provides approximately 210mg of potassium, 220mg of phosphorus, and 52mg of sodium.
- **Cornish Hen:** A type of mini chicken, a 3-ounce serving of cooked Cornish hen has around 230mg of potassium, 190mg of phosphorus, and 61mg of sodium.
- **Crocodile:** An unusual choice, a 3-ounce serving of crocodile contains around 215mg of potassium, 220mg of phosphorus, and 58mg of sodium.
- **Deer:** An excellent game meat, a 3-ounce serving of deer offers approximately 230mg of potassium, 225mg of phosphorus, and 56mg of sodium.
- **Duck Breast:** A prized poultry option, a 3-ounce serving of duck breast provides about 235mg of potassium, 220mg of phosphorus, and 56mg of sodium.
- **Duck Liver:** Rich in flavor, a 3-ounce serving of duck liver has about 230mg of potassium, 320mg of phosphorus, and 57mg of sodium.
- **Duck:** Traditionally rich in flavor, a 3-ounce serving of cooked duck offers approximately 204mg of potassium, 210mg of phosphorus, and 61mg of sodium.
- **Elk:** A game meat lower in fat, a 3-ounce serving of cooked elk has around 241mg of potassium, 178mg of phosphorus, and 57mg of sodium.

- **Emu:** A lean red meat, a 3-ounce serving of cooked emu has around 252mg of potassium, 178mg of phosphorus, and 52mg of sodium.
- **Goat Meat:** A lean red meat, a 3-ounce serving of goat meat provides around 220mg of potassium, 215mg of phosphorus, and 54mg of sodium.
- **Goat:** A popular choice in many cultures, a 3-ounce serving of goat offers about 220mg of potassium, 200mg of phosphorus, and 52mg of sodium.
- **Goose:** Less common but equally nutritious, a 3-ounce serving of cooked goose contains around 252mg of potassium, 215mg of phosphorus, and 63mg of sodium.
- **Guinea Fowl:** A poultry alternative, a 3-ounce serving of cooked guinea fowl provides about 210mg of potassium, 205mg of phosphorus, and 57mg of sodium.
- **Kangaroo:** Lean and gamey, a 3-ounce serving of cooked kangaroo offers approximately 205mg of potassium, 220mg of phosphorus, and 52mg of sodium.
- **Lamb Heart:** Another nutrient-dense choice, a 3-ounce serving of lamb heart provides around 250mg of potassium, 240mg of phosphorus, and 58mg of sodium.
- **Lamb Kidney:** An organ meat, a 3-ounce serving of lamb kidney has approximately 250mg of potassium, 350mg of phosphorus, and 58mg of sodium.
- **Lamb Leg:** A rich choice, a 3-ounce serving of lamb leg contains around 235mg of potassium, 225mg of phosphorus, and 56mg of sodium.
- **Lamb Liver:** A nutrient-dense choice, a 3-ounce serving of lamb liver has around 300mg of potassium, 340mg of phosphorus, and 58mg of sodium.
- **Lamb Loin:** Rich in flavor, a 3-ounce serving of cooked lamb loin provides about 235mg of potassium, 220mg of phosphorus, and 58mg of sodium.
- **Lamb Ribs:** Rich and succulent, a 3-ounce serving of lamb ribs has approximately 235mg of potassium, 210mg of

phosphorus, and 55mg of sodium.

- **Lamb Shank:** A flavorful cut, a 3-ounce serving of cooked lamb shank has approximately 202mg of potassium, 220mg of phosphorus, and 57mg of sodium.
- **Lamb Shoulder:** A tender cut, a 3-ounce serving of lamb shoulder contains approximately 245mg of potassium, 230mg of phosphorus, and 57mg of sodium.
- **Lamb:** A rich source of protein and an occasional treat due to its higher fat content. A 3-ounce serving of cooked lamb has approximately 310mg of potassium, 225mg of phosphorus, and 57mg of sodium.
- **Lean Ground Beef:** Ensure to choose 90% lean; a 3-ounce serving of cooked lean ground beef offers about 248mg of potassium, 186mg of phosphorus, and 55mg of sodium.
- **Lean Ground Chicken:** Ensure to choose 90% lean; a 3-ounce serving of cooked lean ground chicken provides about 240mg of potassium, 190mg of phosphorus, and 53mg of sodium.
- **Lean Ground Lamb:** Ensure to choose 90% lean; a 3-ounce serving of cooked lean ground lamb has approximately 265mg of potassium, 200mg of phosphorus, and 56mg of sodium.
- **Lean Ground Pork:** Ensure to choose 90% lean; a 3-ounce serving of cooked lean ground pork offers about 330mg of potassium, 210mg of phosphorus, and 58mg of sodium.
- **Lean Ground Turkey:** Ensure to choose 90% lean; a 3-ounce serving of cooked lean ground turkey contains around 235mg of potassium, 180mg of phosphorus, and 50mg of sodium.
- **Lean Ground Veal:** Ensure to choose 90% lean; a 3-ounce serving of cooked lean ground veal contains around 250mg of potassium, 215mg of phosphorus, and 53mg of sodium.
- **Lean Ham:** Choose low-sodium varieties; a 3-ounce serving of cooked lean ham offers about 280mg of potassium, 211mg of phosphorus, and 1,200mg of sodium. (Exercise caution due to high sodium)

- **Llama:** A unique meat, a 3-ounce serving of llama contains approximately 235mg of potassium, 220mg of phosphorus, and 55mg of sodium.
- **Moose:** A lean game meat, a 3-ounce serving of cooked moose provides about 220mg of potassium, 210mg of phosphorus, and 50mg of sodium.
- **Mountain Goat:** A game meat, a 3-ounce serving of mountain goat contains around 245mg of potassium, 215mg of phosphorus, and 57mg of sodium.
- **Ostrich:** An unconventional choice, a 3-ounce serving of cooked ostrich offers approximately 254mg of potassium, 190mg of phosphorus, and 54mg of sodium.
- **Partridge:** A small game bird, a 3-ounce serving of partridge offers approximately 215mg of potassium, 210mg of phosphorus, and 52mg of sodium.
- **Peacock:** An unusual choice, a 3-ounce serving of peacock offers around 220mg of potassium, 210mg of phosphorus, and 55mg of sodium.
- **Pheasant:** A classic game bird, a 3-ounce serving of cooked pheasant contains around 254mg of potassium, 232mg of phosphorus, and 58mg of sodium.
- **Pigeon:** A small game bird, a 3-ounce serving of pigeon provides about 215mg of potassium, 240mg of phosphorus, and 55mg of sodium.
- **Pork Belly Ribs:** Flavorful and meaty, a 3-ounce serving of pork belly ribs provides approximately 230mg of potassium, 220mg of phosphorus, and 58mg of sodium.
- **Pork Belly:** Flavorful and fatty, a 3-ounce serving of pork belly provides around 250mg of potassium, 220mg of phosphorus, and 57mg of sodium.
- **Pork Chop:** A popular choice, a 3-ounce serving of pork chop contains approximately 315mg of potassium, 220mg of phosphorus, and 62mg of sodium.
- **Pork Hocks:** A flavorful cut, a 3-ounce serving of pork hocks offers around 225mg of potassium, 220mg of phosphorus,

and 57mg of sodium.

- **Pork Kidney:** An organ meat, a 3-ounce serving of pork kidney contains about 275mg of potassium, 380mg of phosphorus, and 60mg of sodium.
- **Pork Liver:** A less common choice, a 3-ounce serving of pork liver contains around 290mg of potassium, 360mg of phosphorus, and 62mg of sodium.
- **Pork Loin:** A versatile choice, a 3-ounce serving of pork loin provides approximately 240mg of potassium, 225mg of phosphorus, and 54mg of sodium.
- **Pork Loin:** Lean and flavorful, a 3-ounce serving of cooked pork loin provides about 340mg of potassium, 220mg of phosphorus, and 57mg of sodium.
- **Pork Ribs:** Flavorful and tender, a 3-ounce serving of cooked pork ribs contains approximately 250mg of potassium, 215mg of phosphorus, and 58mg of sodium.
- **Pork Shoulder:** A popular cut, a 3-ounce serving of pork shoulder contains about 215mg of potassium, 220mg of phosphorus, and 56mg of sodium.
- **Pork Snout:** A less common choice, a 3-ounce serving of pork snout offers about 210mg of potassium, 210mg of phosphorus, and 58mg of sodium.
- **Pork Tenderloin:** A lean cut, a 3-ounce serving of cooked pork tenderloin contains about 350mg of potassium, 220mg of phosphorus, and 55mg of sodium.
- **Pork Trotters:** Rich in collagen, a 3-ounce serving of pork trotters contains around 210mg of potassium, 220mg of phosphorus, and 59mg of sodium.
- **Pork:** Especially lean cuts like tenderloin. A 3-ounce cooked pork tenderloin offers about 382mg of potassium, 211mg of phosphorus, and 48mg of sodium.
- **Quail:** Small but flavorful, a 3-ounce serving of cooked quail provides about 202mg of potassium, 220mg of phosphorus, and 56mg of sodium.

- **Rabbit:** A lean choice, a 3-ounce serving of rabbit contains around 215mg of potassium, 210mg of phosphorus, and 52mg of sodium.
- **Rabbit:** A less common but lean meat option. A 3-ounce serving of cooked rabbit offers about 204mg of potassium, 214mg of phosphorus, and 47mg of sodium.
- **Raccoon:** Unusual but lean, a 3-ounce serving of raccoon offers approximately 230mg of potassium, 210mg of phosphorus, and 55mg of sodium.
- **Rattlesnake:** A unique choice, a 3-ounce serving of rattlesnake has approximately 200mg of potassium, 210mg of phosphorus, and 52mg of sodium.
- **Snapping Turtle:** A unique choice, a 3-ounce serving of cooked snapping turtle offers about 220mg of potassium, 200mg of phosphorus, and 55mg of sodium.
- **Squab:** A type of pigeon, a 3-ounce serving of squab has approximately 220mg of potassium, 210mg of phosphorus, and 55mg of sodium.
- **Squirrel:** Uncommon but lean, a 3-ounce serving of squirrel has around 200mg of potassium, 230mg of phosphorus, and 50mg of sodium.
- **Turkey Breast:** A lean choice, a 3-ounce serving of turkey breast has around 240mg of potassium, 230mg of phosphorus, and 57mg of sodium.
- **Turkey Neck:** Flavorful and fatty, a 3-ounce serving of turkey neck has approximately 220mg of potassium, 210mg of phosphorus, and 55mg of sodium.
- **Turkey:** Another lean protein source. A 3-ounce serving of cooked turkey breast has around 252mg of potassium, 183mg of phosphorus, and 50mg of sodium.
- **Veal:** Lower in fat compared to many types of meat. A 3-ounce serving of cooked veal contains around 330mg of potassium, 238mg of phosphorus, and 57mg of sodium.
- **Venison Steak:** A lean game meat, a 3-ounce serving of cooked venison steak has approximately 245mg of

potassium, 215mg of phosphorus, and 55mg of sodium.

- **Venison:** Another game meat, a 3-ounce serving of venison provides approximately 240mg of potassium, 230mg of phosphorus, and 56mg of sodium.
- **Venison:** High in protein and lower in fat, a 3-ounce serving of cooked venison provides around 248mg of potassium, 192mg of phosphorus, and 62mg of sodium.
- **Wild Boar:** Gamey in flavor, a 3-ounce serving of cooked wild boar contains approximately 220mg of potassium, 210mg of phosphorus, and 58mg of sodium.
- **Wild Rabbit:** Lean and gamey, a 3-ounce serving of wild rabbit has approximately 210mg of potassium, 215mg of phosphorus, and 50mg of sodium.

As with any food, meats should be eaten in moderation to maintain balanced potassium, phosphorus, and sodium levels. Lean options like chicken or turkey are generally safe for individuals with kidney disease but always monitor portion sizes. Higher-fat meats like lamb should be occasional treats. Consider your dietary needs and consult your healthcare provider for personalized advice. These meats are usually good choices for a kidney-friendly diet, but everyone's body is unique, and food reactions can vary. Regular monitoring and consultation with your healthcare provider or dietitian is vital.

When selecting lean meats, it's important to understand what to look for. Lean meats have less than 10 grams of total fat, 4.5 grams or less of saturated fat, and less than 95 milligrams of cholesterol per 3.5 ounces (100 grams). Poultry, such as chicken and turkey, especially the breasts, are often lean cuts. In red meats, look for cuts with the words "loin" or "round" in the name, as these are typically leaner. Game meats like venison and elk are generally leaner than domestic meats.

Controlling portion size is also crucial in a balanced diet. A single serving of meat is typically 3 ounces, about the size of a deck of cards or the palm of your hand. Avoid eating large quantities of meat in one sitting, as this can lead to overconsumption of calories, fat, and cholesterol, potentially leading to health issues over time.

It's also beneficial to be mindful of the cooking methods. Grilling, broiling, roasting, steaming, or boiling meats without adding fat can help keep your meats leaner. Avoid frying or sautéing in large amounts of fat and remove any visible fat before cooking.

Finally, remember that while lean meats are a great source of protein, they're just one piece of the dietary puzzle. Balance your diet with plenty of fruits, vegetables, whole grains, and low-fat dairy to ensure a wide range of nutrients. Always consult a healthcare professional or dietitian for advice tailored to your nutritional needs.

4.12. Nuts and Seeds

Potassium: Individuals with kidney disease are often advised to restrict their daily potassium intake to approximately 2,000 milligrams (mg). Excessive potassium can lead to a serious condition called hyperkalemia, which can disrupt heart rhythm.

Phosphorus: People with kidney disease are generally recommended to limit their daily phosphorus consumption to around 800-1,000 mg. Elevated phosphorus levels can contribute to long-term bone and heart problems.

Sodium: For those with kidney disease, it is generally advised to limit daily sodium intake to less than 2,000 mg. A high-sodium diet can result in fluid retention and high blood pressure, further compromising kidney health.

- **Almonds:** A handful (about 24 nuts) of almonds contains approximately 208mg of potassium, 134mg of phosphorus, and 1mg of sodium. They are a great source of healthy fats and dietary fiber.
- **Apricot Seeds:** A 1-ounce serving of apricot seeds offers around 150mg of potassium, 60mg of phosphorus, and no

sodium. Apricot seeds are a good source of dietary fiber and monounsaturated fats.

- **Beech Nuts:** A 1-ounce serving of beech nuts offers approximately 220mg of potassium, 145mg of phosphorus, and no sodium. Beech nuts are rich in protein and beneficial fats.
- **Black Walnuts:** A 1-ounce serving of black walnuts contains approximately 155mg of potassium, 85mg of phosphorus, and 2mg of sodium. Black walnuts are a good source of heart-healthy fats.
- **Brazil Nuts:** A 1-ounce serving of Brazil nuts contains approximately 187mg of potassium, 205mg of phosphorus, and 1mg of sodium. Brazil nuts are notably high in selenium.
- **Cashews:** A 1-ounce serving of cashews contains about 160mg of potassium, 168mg of phosphorus, and 3mg of sodium. Cashews are a good source of magnesium and have a rich, buttery taste.
- **Chestnuts:** A 1-ounce serving of chestnuts contains about 168mg of potassium, 29mg of phosphorus, and 1mg of sodium. Chestnuts are high in fiber and have low-fat content compared to other nuts.
- **Chia Seeds:** A tablespoon of chia seeds contains about 45mg of potassium, 65mg of phosphorus, and 1mg of sodium. Chia seeds are high in fiber and can be easily added to many dishes.
- **Coconut (dried):** A 1-ounce serving of dried coconut contains approximately 160mg of potassium, 90mg of phosphorus, and 5mg of sodium. Dried coconut is a good source of fiber and beneficial fats.
- **Flaxseeds:** A tablespoon provides around 83mg of potassium, 65mg of phosphorus, and 2mg of sodium. They are a great source of Omega-3 fatty acids.
- **Ginkgo Nuts:** A 1-ounce serving of ginkgo nuts contains approximately 510mg of potassium, 10mg of phosphorus,

and 15mg of sodium. Ginkgo nuts are a good source of dietary fiber and antioxidants.

- **Hazel Pine Nut:** A 1-ounce serving of hazel pine nut contains about 180mg of potassium, 110mg of phosphorus, and 1mg of sodium. Hazel pine nuts are a good source of monounsaturated fats and fiber.
- **Hazelnuts:** A 1-ounce serving of hazelnuts offers approximately 192mg of potassium, 86mg of phosphorus, and 1mg of sodium. Hazelnuts are high in Vitamin E and have a distinctive sweet flavor.
- **Hemp Seeds:** A tablespoon of hemp seeds provides about 170mg of potassium, 165mg of phosphorus, and 1mg of sodium. They are a great source of plant-based protein.
- **Lotus Seeds:** A 1-ounce serving of lotus seeds offers around 350mg of potassium, 96mg of phosphorus, and 1mg of sodium. Lotus seeds are a good source of protein and low in fat.
- **Macadamia Nuts:** A 1-ounce serving of macadamia nuts has around 103mg of potassium, 53mg of phosphorus, and 1mg of sodium. They are rich in healthy fats and have a creamy taste.
- **Mamoncillo Nuts:** A 1-ounce serving of mamoncillo nuts provides around 240mg of potassium, 80mg of phosphorus, and no sodium. Mamoncillo nuts are a good source of dietary fiber and antioxidants.
- **Peanuts:** A 1-ounce serving of peanuts provides approximately 200mg of potassium, 101mg of phosphorus, and 2mg of sodium. They are a great source of monounsaturated fats and protein.
- **Pecans:** A 1-ounce serving (about 19 halves) of pecans provides approximately 116mg of potassium, 48mg of phosphorus, and just 1mg of sodium. Pecans are rich in monounsaturated fats, which are good for heart health.
- **Pili Nuts:** A 1-ounce serving of pili nuts provides approximately 200mg of potassium, 60mg of phosphorus,

and no sodium. Pili nuts are a good source of healthy fats and protein.

- **Pine Nuts:** A 1-ounce serving of pine nuts provides about 169mg of potassium, 163mg of phosphorus, and 1mg of sodium. They are a good source of Vitamin K.
- **Pistachios:** A 1-ounce serving (around 49 nuts) of pistachios contains approximately 291mg of potassium, 137mg of phosphorus, and 1mg of sodium. Pistachios are rich in fiber and may aid in weight loss.
- **Poppy Seeds:** A tablespoon of poppy seeds contains approximately 70mg of potassium, 79mg of phosphorus, and 1mg of sodium. Poppy seeds are high in fiber and can be easily incorporated into various dishes.
- **Pumpkin Seeds:** A 1-ounce serving of pumpkin seeds provides about 261mg of potassium, 332mg of phosphorus, and 5mg of sodium. Pumpkin seeds are beneficial for prostate health.
- **Sesame Seeds:** A tablespoon of sesame seeds contains approximately 57mg of potassium, 57mg of phosphorus, and 1mg of sodium. They are a great source of various minerals like magnesium and zinc.
- **Sunflower Seeds:** A 1-ounce serving of sunflower seeds offers approximately 241mg of potassium, 227mg of phosphorus, and 1mg of sodium. These seeds are high in Vitamin E and selenium.
- **Tiger nuts:** A 1-ounce serving of tiger nuts provides about 215mg of potassium, 115mg of phosphorus, and 5mg of sodium. Tiger nuts are fiber-rich, making them a good choice for digestive health.
- **Walnuts:** 14 halves provide about 125mg of potassium, 98mg of phosphorus, and 1mg of sodium. They are high in antioxidants and beneficial for heart health.
- **Watermelon Seeds:** A 1-ounce serving of watermelon seeds provides about 146mg of potassium, 82mg of phosphorus,

and 3mg of sodium. Watermelon seeds are rich in magnesium and iron.

Please note that portion control is essential when consuming nuts and seeds as they can be high in phosphorus. It's also important to choose unsalted varieties to keep your sodium intake in check. Regular monitoring and consultation with your healthcare provider or dietitian is vital.

Incorporating nuts and seeds into a kidney-friendly diet can confer several health benefits, if portion control is properly observed. These superfoods are packed with essential vitamins, minerals, antioxidants, and heart-healthy fats, which are known to support overall health, including kidney function.

Firstly, the high content of antioxidants in nuts and seeds helps fight oxidative stress, a condition linked to kidney damage. By scavenging harmful free radicals in the body, antioxidants protect kidney cells and support their repair and regeneration.

Secondly, the rich fiber content found in these foods contributes to digestive health. It helps regulate blood glucose and cholesterol levels, which are crucial for those with kidney-related issues. Maintaining stable blood sugar and cholesterol levels can prevent further kidney damage in chronic kidney disease patients.

Thirdly, unsaturated fats found in generous amounts in nuts and seeds have been found to reduce inflammation, a common complication in those with kidney disease. By reducing inflammation, these heart-healthy fats can help slow the progression of kidney disease.

Lastly, while nuts and seeds do contain phosphorus, a mineral that needs to be monitored in a kidney-friendly diet, it's important to note that only about 40-60% of the phosphorus in nuts, seeds, and legumes is absorbed by the body, thanks to phytic acid, which inhibits phosphorus absorption.

However, despite these advantages, nuts and seeds are calorie-dense foods, so they should be consumed in moderation. Overeating these foods can lead to weight gain and increased phosphorus levels. Hence, it's essential to practice portion control and regularly consult with a healthcare provider or dietitian to ensure optimal health outcomes.

4.13. Spices and Herbs

Potassium: Individuals with kidney disease are often recommended to restrict their daily potassium intake to approximately 2,000 milligrams (mg). Excessive potassium can lead to a serious condition known as hyperkalemia, which can disrupt heart rhythm.

Phosphorus: People with kidney disease are generally advised to limit their daily phosphorus consumption to around 800-1,000 mg. Elevated phosphorus levels can contribute to long-term bone and heart complications.

Sodium: It is generally advised for those with kidney disease to limit daily sodium intake to less than 2,000 mg. A high-sodium diet can result in fluid retention and high blood pressure, further compromising kidney health.

- **Allspice:** A teaspoon offers 10mg of potassium, 2mg of phosphorus, and no sodium. Allspice is commonly used in baking and Caribbean cuisine.
- **Basil:** A teaspoon of dried basil contains around 27mg of potassium, 2mg of phosphorus, and zero sodium. This aromatic herb is a great way to enhance the flavor of dishes without adding extra sodium.
- **Bay Leaves:** A single bay leaf offers 4mg of potassium, 2mg of phosphorus, and no sodium. Bay leaves are often used in soups, stews, and other slow-cooked dishes.
- **Black Pepper:** A teaspoon of black pepper provides 37mg of potassium, 10mg of phosphorus, and 1mg of sodium. Black

pepper is a versatile spice that can be used in nearly any dish.

- **Black Sesame Seeds:** A teaspoon of black sesame seeds provides 35mg of potassium, 7mg of phosphorus, and 1mg of sodium. Black sesame seeds are often used in Asian and Middle Eastern cuisines.
- **Caraway Seeds:** A teaspoon of caraway seeds contains 20mg of potassium, 7mg of phosphorus, and no sodium. Caraway seeds are often used in European and Middle Eastern dishes.
- **Cardamom:** A teaspoon of cardamom offers 68mg of potassium, 10mg of phosphorus, and 1mg of sodium. Cardamom is commonly used in Indian and Middle Eastern cuisine.
- **Carob Powder:** A tablespoon of carob powder contains 92mg of potassium, 3mg of phosphorus, and 4mg of sodium. Carob powder is often used as a cocoa substitute in baking.
- **Carom Seeds:** A teaspoon of carom seeds delivers 43mg of potassium, 7mg of phosphorus, and 3mg of sodium. Carom seeds are used in Indian and Middle Eastern cuisines.
- **Cayenne Pepper:** A teaspoon of cayenne pepper contains 30mg of potassium, 3mg of phosphorus, and 1mg of sodium. Cayenne pepper can be used to add heat to a variety of dishes.
- **Celery Seeds:** A teaspoon of celery seeds provides 33mg of potassium, 9mg of phosphorus, and 3mg of sodium. Celery seeds are often used in pickling and coleslaw recipes.
- **Chili Powder:** A teaspoon of chili powder contains 43mg of potassium, 9mg of phosphorus, and 4mg of sodium. Chili powder is great for adding flavor and heat to various dishes.
- **Chives:** A tablespoon of fresh chives contains 16mg of potassium, 2mg of phosphorus, and 1mg of sodium. Chives are great in salads, baked potatoes, and other savory dishes.
- **Cilantro:** A teaspoon of dried cilantro offers 1mg of potassium, zero phosphorus, and zero sodium. Cilantro can be used in salsas, marinades, and Asian dishes.

- **Cinnamon:** A teaspoon of cinnamon offers 11mg of potassium, 2mg of phosphorus, and 0mg of sodium. Cinnamon is commonly used in sweet and savory dishes.
- **Cloves:** A teaspoon of cloves provides 21mg of potassium, 8mg of phosphorus, and 5mg of sodium. Cloves can be used in baking, cooking, and drinks.
- **Cocoa Powder:** A tablespoon of unsweetened cocoa powder offers 131mg of potassium, 27mg of phosphorus, and 1mg of sodium. Cocoa powder is used in a variety of desserts and beverages.
- **Coriander:** A teaspoon of coriander offers 35mg of potassium, 7mg of phosphorus, and 2mg of sodium. Coriander can be used in various dishes, from soups to curries.
- **Cumin:** A teaspoon of cumin provides 22mg of potassium, 7mg of phosphorus, and 10mg of sodium. Cumin is a staple in many Mexican, Middle Eastern, and Indian dishes.
- **Dill:** A tablespoon of fresh dill contains 21mg of potassium, 2mg of phosphorus, and 2mg of sodium. Dill can be used in salads, dips, and fish dishes.
- **Fennel Seeds:** A teaspoon of fennel seeds contains 23mg of potassium, 8mg of phosphorus, and 5mg of sodium. Fennel seeds are often used in Italian and Indian dishes.
- **Fenugreek:** A teaspoon of fenugreek provides 7mg of potassium, 1mg of phosphorus, and no sodium. Fenugreek is commonly used in Indian and Middle Eastern cuisines.
- **Garam Masala:** A teaspoon of garam masala delivers 12mg of potassium, 4mg of phosphorus, and 3mg of sodium. Garam masala is a blend of spices often used in Indian cuisine.
- **Garlic Powder:** A teaspoon of garlic powder offers 26mg of potassium, 14mg of phosphorus, and 1mg of sodium. Garlic Powder is a versatile spice that can be used in a wide array of dishes to boost flavor.

- **Ginger:** A teaspoon of ground ginger contains 8mg of potassium, 1mg of phosphorus, and 1mg of sodium. Ginger can be used in Asian dishes, teas, and desserts.
- **Horseradish:** A teaspoon of horseradish contains 12mg of potassium, 4mg of phosphorus, and no sodium. Horseradish adds a spicy kick to sauces and meats.
- **Juniper Berries:** A teaspoon of juniper berries offers 5mg of potassium, 1mg of phosphorus, and no sodium. Juniper berries are often used in Scandinavian and European cuisines.
- **Lemongrass:** A teaspoon of lemongrass provides 5mg of potassium, 0mg of phosphorus, and no sodium. Lemongrass is a key ingredient in Thai and Vietnamese cuisines.
- **Marjoram:** A teaspoon of marjoram delivers 8mg of potassium, 0mg of phosphorus, and no sodium. Marjoram is often used in Mediterranean cuisine.
- **Mint:** A tablespoon of fresh mint provides 18mg of potassium, 1mg of phosphorus, and zero sodium. Mint is often used in desserts, drinks, and Middle Eastern dishes.
- **Mustard Seeds:** A teaspoon of mustard seeds provides 22mg of potassium, 9mg of phosphorus, and no sodium. Mustard seeds are a common ingredient in Indian cooking.
- **Nutmeg:** A teaspoon of nutmeg contains 7mg of potassium, 0mg of phosphorus, and 0mg of sodium. Nutmeg is often used in baked goods and beverages.
- **Onion Powder:** A teaspoon of onion powder provides 24mg of potassium, 4mg of phosphorus, and 2mg of sodium. Onion powder can enhance the flavor of meats, soups, and stews.
- **Oregano:** A teaspoon of oregano contains 8mg of potassium, 3mg of phosphorus, and no sodium. Oregano is commonly used in Italian and Mediterranean dishes.
- **Paprika:** A teaspoon of paprika provides 37mg of potassium, 7mg of phosphorus, and 2mg of sodium. Paprika is often used in Hungarian cuisine and barbecue dishes.

- **Parsley:** A tablespoon of fresh parsley provides 4mg of potassium, 1mg of phosphorus, and 1mg of sodium. Parsley is a versatile herb that can be added to salads, soups, and stews.
- **Rosemary:** A teaspoon of dried rosemary has approximately 11mg of potassium, 4mg of phosphorus, and zero sodium. Rosemary can be used to flavor meats and vegetables.
- **Saffron:** A teaspoon of saffron contains 2mg of potassium, 1mg of phosphorus, and no sodium. Saffron is a luxurious spice used in Mediterranean and Middle Eastern cuisines.
- **Sage:** A teaspoon of sage contains 4mg of potassium, 0mg of phosphorus, and 0mg of sodium. Sage is commonly used in poultry dishes and stuffing.
- **Star Anise:** A teaspoon of star anise offers 10mg of potassium, 5mg of phosphorus, and 1mg of sodium. Star anise can be used in baking, cooking, and drinks.
- **Tarragon:** A teaspoon of tarragon provides 3mg of potassium, 1mg of phosphorus, and no sodium. Tarragon is a fundamental ingredient in French cuisine.
- **Thyme:** A teaspoon of dried thyme offers 5mg of potassium, 3mg of phosphorus, and zero sodium. Thyme can be a great addition to soups, stews, and meats.
- **Turmeric:** A teaspoon of turmeric contains 64mg of potassium, 7mg of phosphorus, and 1mg of sodium. Turmeric is often used in Indian dishes and has potent anti-inflammatory properties.
- **White Sesame Seeds:** A teaspoon of white sesame seeds offers 39mg of potassium, 7mg of phosphorus, and 1mg of sodium. White sesame seeds are used in a variety of dishes worldwide.

Remember to use these spices and herbs to enhance the flavor of foods while keeping your potassium, phosphorus, and sodium intake in check. Always choose fresh or dried herbs over salted ones to maintain a kidney-friendly diet.

Incorporating flavor into a kidney-friendly diet can be challenging due to the need to limit sodium, potassium, and phosphorus intake. However, various low-sodium and low-potassium alternatives can enhance the taste of your meals without compromising kidney health.

Vinegar, such as balsamic, apple cider, or red wine vinegar, can add a tangy flavor to salads, vegetables, and marinades. **Lemon or lime juice** can bring a fresh zest to fish, chicken, or vegetable dishes, but be mindful of the potassium content if you're on a strict potassium diet.

Herb and spice blends made without salt, like Mrs. Dash or McCormick's Salt-Free blends, can significantly enhance the flavor profile of various dishes.

Fresh or dried herbs offer flavor without additional sodium or potassium. For a Mexican twist, experiment with combinations like basil and oregano for an Italian flare or cilantro and lime.

Low-sodium broths can be used to make soups or stews, as a marinade, or as a cooking medium for grains like rice and quinoa to add flavor without potassium or sodium.

Homemade salsa can be a great way to add flavor to various dishes. You can make a simple salsa using fresh tomatoes, onions, and vinegar.

Everyone's dietary needs and tastes are different, so it's important to consult with your healthcare provider or dietitian about which foods and flavors are right for you.

4.14. Vegetables and Vegetables Products

Potassium: People with kidney disease are often advised to limit their daily potassium intake to around 2,000 milligrams (mg). Too much potassium can cause a serious condition called hyperkalemia, which can affect heart rhythm.

Phosphorus: Individuals with kidney disease are generally recommended to restrict their daily phosphorus consumption to approximately 800-1,000 mg. Elevated phosphorus levels can contribute to long-term complications in the bones and heart.

Sodium: It is generally recommended for those with kidney disease to limit daily sodium intake to less than 2,000 mg. A high-sodium diet can cause fluid retention and high blood pressure, which can further harm kidney health.

- **Apples:** One medium apple has around 195mg of potassium, 10mg of phosphorus, and 2mg of sodium. Apples are high in fiber and vitamin C.
- **Apricots:** One medium apricot contains approximately 173mg of potassium, 13mg of phosphorus, and 1mg of sodium. Apricots are a good source of vitamins A and C.
- **Artichokes:** A medium-sized, cooked artichoke contains approximately 343mg of potassium, 89mg of phosphorus, and 70mg of sodium. Artichokes are a good source of fiber, vitamin C, and folate.
- **Arugula:** One cup contains approximately 74mg of potassium, 15mg of phosphorus, and 5mg of sodium. Arugula is rich in vitamins A and K.
- **Asparagus:** A half-cup of cooked asparagus offers around 202mg of potassium, 32mg of phosphorus, and 13mg of sodium. Asparagus is a good source of fiber, folate, and vitamins A, C, and K.
- **Avocados:** Half of a medium avocado provides around 487mg of potassium, 30mg of phosphorus, and 5mg of sodium. Avocados are packed with heart-healthy monounsaturated fats and fiber.
- **Bananas:** A medium banana contains approximately 422mg of potassium, 26mg of phosphorus, and 1mg of sodium. Bananas are known for their high potassium content and are a great vitamin C and B6 source.

- **Beets:** A half-cup of boiled, sliced beets offers around 259mg of potassium, 32mg of phosphorus, and 64mg of sodium. Beets are a good source of folate and provide a good amount of fiber.
- **Bell Peppers:** A half-cup of chopped bell peppers provides about 152mg of potassium, 13mg of phosphorus, and 1mg of sodium. Bell peppers are a colorful dish with addition high in vitamins C and B6.
- **Black Beans:** One cup of cooked black beans contains approximately 611mg of potassium, 241mg of phosphorus, and 1mg of sodium. Black beans are rich in fiber and protein.
- **Blackberries:** A half-cup offers around 117mg of potassium, 15mg of phosphorus, and 1mg of sodium. Blackberries are high in fiber and rich in antioxidants.
- **Blueberries:** A half-cup offers around 57mg of potassium, 6mg of phosphorus, and 1mg of sodium. Blueberries are antioxidant-rich and high in fiber and vitamin C.
- **Bok Choy:** One cup of cooked bok choy provides about 631mg of potassium, 45mg of phosphorus, and 57mg of sodium. Bok Choy is a great source of vitamins A and C.
- **Broccoli:** A half-cup of boiled broccoli contains approximately 144mg of potassium, 29mg of phosphorus, and 20mg of sodium. Broccoli is a powerhouse of nutrients, including Vitamin K, Vitamin C, and dietary fiber.
- **Brussels sprouts:** A half-cup of cooked Brussels sprouts provides about 247mg of potassium, 32mg of phosphorus, and 16mg of sodium. Brussels sprouts are a powerhouse of nutrients, high in fiber and vitamins C and K.
- **Cabbage:** A half-cup of cooked cabbage contains approximately 147mg of potassium, 16mg of phosphorus, and 12mg of sodium. Cabbage is rich in vitamins C and K and is beneficial for heart health.
- **Cantaloupes:** A half-cup of cubed cantaloupes contains about 214mg of potassium, 7mg of phosphorus, and 14mg of sodium. Cantaloupes are a refreshing and nutritious

fruit with high water content and are rich in vitamins A
and C.

- **Carrots:** A medium-sized raw carrot provides about 195mg of
  potassium, 25mg of phosphorus, and 42mg of sodium.
  Carrots are known for their beta-carotene content, converted
  to Vitamin A in the body.
- **Cauliflower:** One cup of cooked cauliflower contains
  approximately 176mg of potassium, 40mg of phosphorus,
  and 19mg of sodium. Cauliflower is high in vitamins C and K.
- **Celery:** A medium stalk of celery offers around 104mg of
  potassium, 11mg of phosphorus, and 32mg of sodium. Celery
  is crisp and refreshing, perfect for snacking or adding to
  salads and stir-fries.
- **Chard:** A cup of cooked chard provides about 961mg of
  potassium, 58mg of phosphorus, and 313mg of sodium.
  Chard is rich in vitamins A and K.
- **Cherries:** A half-cup of cherries provides about 134mg of
  potassium, 10mg of phosphorus, and 0mg of sodium.
  Cherries are packed with antioxidants and anti-
  inflammatory compounds.
- **Chickpeas:** One cup of cooked chickpeas contains
  approximately 477mg of potassium, 276mg of phosphorus,
  and 11mg of sodium. Chickpeas are high in fiber and a good
  source of protein.
- **Cilantro:** One cup of chopped cilantro provides about 521mg
  of potassium, 37mg of phosphorus, and 46mg of sodium.
  Cilantro is a good source of vitamins A and K.
- **Collard Greens:** One cup of cooked collard greens offers
  around 220mg of potassium, 25mg of phosphorus, and 30mg
  of sodium. Collard greens are high in vitamins A and K.
- **Corn:** A half-cup of cooked corn offers around 168mg of
  potassium, 42mg of phosphorus, and 6mg of sodium. Corn is
  a versatile vegetable that can be used in various dishes.
- **Cucumbers:** A half-cup of sliced cucumber contains around
  76mg of potassium, 11mg of phosphorus, and 1mg of sodium.

Cucumbers are refreshing and hydrating, perfect for salads and sandwiches.

- **Edamame:** One cup of cooked edamame provides about 676mg of potassium, 262mg of phosphorus, and 9mg of sodium. Edamame is rich in protein and fiber.
- **Eggplant:** A half-cup of cooked eggplant contains about 122mg of potassium, 12mg of phosphorus, and 1mg of sodium. Eggplant is a versatile vegetable that can be roasted, grilled, or baked.
- **Endive:** One cup of chopped endive offers around 157mg of potassium, 15mg of phosphorus, and 11mg of sodium. Endive is a good source of vitamins A and C.
- **Escarole:** A cup of cooked escarole provides about 218mg of potassium, 40mg of phosphorus, and 2mg of sodium. Escarole is rich in vitamins A and K.
- **Fennel:** One medium bulb offers around 963mg of potassium, 115mg of phosphorus, and 124mg of sodium. Fennel is high in vitamin C.
- **Figs:** One medium fig contains approximately 92mg of potassium, 14mg of phosphorus, and 1mg of sodium. Figs are high in fiber and a good source of several essential minerals.
- **Garlic:** A half-clove of garlic has around 12mg of potassium, 4mg of phosphorus, and 1mg of sodium. Garlic not only adds flavor to dishes but also offers potential health benefits, such as boosting immunity and reducing blood pressure.
- **Ginger:** A half-inch piece of fresh ginger contains approximately 23mg of potassium, 2mg of phosphorus, and 0mg of sodium. Ginger is a popular spice used in cooking and also has anti-inflammatory properties.
- **Grapefruit:** One medium grapefruit provides around 166mg of potassium, 18mg of phosphorus, and 0mg of sodium. Grapefruits are a fantastic source of antioxidants and vitamin C.
- **Grapes:** A half-cup of grapes contains about 144mg of potassium, 7mg of phosphorus, and 1mg of sodium. Grapes

come in many varieties and are a great source of
antioxidants.

- **Green Beans:** A half cup of raw green beans has around
  88mg of potassium, 21mg of phosphorus, and 3mg of sodium.
  Green beans can be a great meal addition, providing fiber
  and vitamin C.
- **Green Peas:** A half-cup of cooked green peas provides about
  187mg of potassium, 87mg of phosphorus, and 5mg of
  sodium. Green peas are a good source of vitamins A, C,
  and K.
- **Horseradish:** One tablespoon of prepared horseradish
  contains approximately 44mg of potassium, 8mg of
  phosphorus, and 47mg of sodium. Horseradish is a good
  source of vitamin C.
- **Kale:** One cup of chopped kale provides about 329mg of
  potassium, 37mg of phosphorus, and 29mg of sodium. Kale is
  highly nutritious, loaded with antioxidants, and an excellent
  source of vitamins A, C, and K.
- **Kidney Beans:** One cup of cooked kidney beans offers
  around 713mg of potassium, 263mg of phosphorus, and 2mg
  of sodium. Kidney beans are high in fiber and a good source
  of protein.
- **Kiwi:** One medium kiwi offers around 215mg of potassium,
  20mg of phosphorus, and 3mg of sodium. Kiwis are rich in
  vitamins C and E and high in fiber.
- **Kohlrabi:** One cup of raw kohlrabi provides about 473mg of
  potassium, 62mg of phosphorus, and 27mg of sodium.
  Kohlrabi is high in vitamins A and C.
- **Leeks:** One cup of sliced leeks offers around 160mg of
  potassium, 42mg of phosphorus, and 18mg of sodium. Leeks
  are a good source of vitamin A and provide a subtle, sweet
  flavor.
- **Lentils:** One cup of cooked lentils provides about 731mg of
  potassium, 365mg of phosphorus, and 4mg of sodium.
  Lentils are packed with fiber and protein.

- **Lettuce:** One cup of shredded iceberg contains about 102mg of potassium, 10mg of phosphorus, and 3mg of sodium. Lettuce is a salad staple that provides a good amount of vitamin K.
- **Lima Beans:** One cup of cooked lima beans offers around 955mg of potassium, 209mg of phosphorus, and 5mg of sodium. Lima beans are a great source of dietary fiber and protein.
- **Limes:** One medium lime contains approximately 68mg of potassium, 6mg of phosphorus, and 1mg of sodium. Limes are a good source of vitamin C and antioxidants.
- **Mangoes:** One cup of sliced mango provides about 277mg of potassium, 18mg of phosphorus, and 3mg of sodium. Mangoes are a great source of vitamins A and C and are fiber rich.
- **Mushrooms:** A half-cup of cooked white mushrooms offers around 223mg of potassium, 42mg of phosphorus, and 3mg of sodium. Mushrooms are a low-calorie option for adding flavor and texture to dishes.
- **Mustard Greens:** One cup of cooked mustard greens offers around 284mg of potassium, 58mg of phosphorus, and 18mg of sodium. Mustard greens are high in vitamins A and K.
- **Navy Beans:** One cup of cooked navy beans provides about 708mg of potassium, 255mg of phosphorus, and 2mg of sodium. Navy beans are a good source of fiber and protein.
- **Olives:** A half-cup of sliced olives provides about 4mg of potassium, 0mg of phosphorus, and 735mg of sodium. Olives are high in healthy fats and vitamin E.
- **Onions:** A half-cup of chopped onions contains approximately 116mg of potassium, 12mg of phosphorus, and 1mg of sodium. Onions are a staple in many cuisines and provide good vitamin C.
- **Oranges:** A medium orange contains approximately 237mg of potassium, 18mg of phosphorus, and 1mg of sodium. Oranges are famous for their vitamin C content.

- **Papayas:** One medium papaya provides about 781mg of potassium, 61mg of phosphorus, and 30mg of sodium. Papayas are a good source of antioxidants and are rich in vitamin C.
- **Parsley:** One cup of chopped parsley contains approximately 332mg of potassium, 34mg of phosphorus, and 34mg of sodium. Parsley is a good source of vitamins A, C, and K.
- **Parsnips:** One medium parsnip contains approximately 573mg of potassium, 90mg of phosphorus, and 13mg of sodium. Parsnips are rich in vitamin C and fiber.
- **Peaches:** A medium peach contains approximately 285mg of potassium, 20mg of phosphorus, and 0mg of sodium. Peaches are good sources of vitamins A, C, and potassium.
- **Pears:** A medium pear provides around 206mg of potassium, 16mg of phosphorus, and 1mg of sodium. Pears are a great source of dietary fiber and vitamin C.
- **Peas:** A half-cup of cooked green peas contains approximately 178mg of potassium, 53mg of phosphorus, and 4mg of sodium. Peas are a good source of fiber, protein, and vitamins A, C, and K.
- **Peppers:** A half-cup of sliced bell peppers offers approximately 117mg of potassium, 11mg of phosphorus, and 2mg of sodium. Peppers are high in vitamins A and C.
- **Pineapple:** A half-cup of pineapple offers around 89mg of potassium, 6mg of phosphorus, and 1mg of sodium. Pineapple is a tropical fruit rich in vitamins, enzymes, and antioxidants.
- **Pinto Beans:** One cup of cooked pinto beans offers around 746mg of potassium, 251mg of phosphorus, and 1mg of sodium. Pinto beans are high in fiber and a good source of protein.
- **Plums:** One medium plum offer around 104mg of potassium, 12mg of phosphorus, and 0mg of sodium. Plums are high in antioxidants, helping to reduce inflammation and protect against chronic disease.

- **Pomegranates:** One pomegranate offers around 666mg of potassium, 102mg of phosphorus, and 8mg of sodium. Pomegranates are packed with antioxidants and are high in fiber and vitamin C.
- **Potatoes:** One medium baked potato provides about 941mg of potassium, 129mg of phosphorus, and 17mg of sodium. Potatoes are a good source of vitamin C.
- **Pumpkin:** A half-cup of cooked, mashed pumpkin contains about 240mg of potassium, 22mg of phosphorus, and 1mg of sodium. Pumpkin is rich in vitamin A and provides a good amount of fiber.
- **Radicchio:** A cup of shredded radicchio provides about 121mg of potassium, 16mg of phosphorus, and 9mg of sodium. Radicchio is a good source of vitamin K.
- **Radishes:** A half-cup of sliced radishes offers around 135mg of potassium, 12mg of phosphorus, and 23mg of sodium. Radishes add a punch of flavor to salads and side dishes and offer health benefits, such as aiding digestion and reducing the risk of heart disease.
- **Raspberries:** A half-cup offers around 93mg of potassium, 15mg of phosphorus, and 1mg of sodium. Raspberries are a fantastic source of fiber and vitamin C.
- **Red bell peppers:** A half-cup of red bell peppers contains around 88mg of potassium, 10mg of phosphorus, and 1mg of sodium. Red bell peppers are rich in vitamin C and contain antioxidants A and B6. They also possess a lower amount of potassium compared to other vegetables.
- **Red Peppers:** One medium red pepper provides about 251mg of potassium, 29mg of phosphorus, and 3mg of sodium. Red peppers are high in vitamins A and C.
- **Rhubarb:** One cup of diced rhubarb offers around 351mg of potassium, 105mg of phosphorus, and 5mg of sodium. Rhubarb is high in vitamin K and a good source of calcium.
- **Romaine Lettuce:** One cup of shredded romaine lettuce contains approximately 116mg of potassium, 20mg of

phosphorus, and 4mg of sodium. Romaine lettuce is a good source of vitamins A and K.

- **Rutabaga:** One medium rutabaga contains approximately 782mg of potassium, 120mg of phosphorus, and 28mg of sodium. Rutabagas are high in vitamin C and fiber.
- **Soybeans:** One cup of cooked soybeans provides about 886mg of potassium, 515mg of phosphorus, and 1mg of sodium. Soybeans are high in protein and fiber.
- **Spinach:** A half-cup of boiled spinach offers around 420mg of potassium, 49mg of phosphorus, and 63mg of sodium. Spinach is a leafy green rich in vitamins A, C, and K, iron, and calcium.
- **Squash:** One cup of cooked squash contains approximately 494mg of potassium, 82mg of phosphorus, and 2mg of sodium. Squash is high in vitamins A and C.
- **Strawberries:** A half-cup of strawberries contains about 139mg of potassium, 16mg of phosphorus, and 1mg of sodium. Strawberries are an excellent source of vitamin C and manganese.
- **Sweet Potatoes:** A medium-sized baked sweet potato contains approximately 542mg of potassium, 74mg of phosphorus, and 41mg of sodium. Sweet potatoes are packed with vitamin A and provide good fiber.
- **Swiss Chard:** A half-cup of boiled Swiss chard has around 480mg of potassium, 32mg of phosphorus, and 313mg of sodium. Swiss chard is a leafy green rich in vitamins A, C, and K.
- **Tempeh:** One cup of cooked tempeh contains approximately 684mg of potassium, 411mg of phosphorus, and 15mg of sodium. Tempeh is high in protein and a good source of iron.
- **Tofu:** A half-cup of firm tofu offers around 150mg of potassium, 138mg of phosphorus, and 10mg of sodium. Tofu is a good source of protein and calcium.

- **Tomatoes:** A medium-sized raw tomato contains approximately 292mg of potassium, 24mg of phosphorus, and 5mg of sodium. Tomatoes are a good source of vitamins A, C, and K and the antioxidant lycopene.
- **Turnips:** A half-cup of boiled, cubed turnips contains around 127mg of potassium, 20mg of phosphorus, and 12mg of sodium. They can be used instead of potatoes in some recipes and offer less potassium.
- **Watercress:** One cup of raw watercress contains approximately 112mg of potassium, 15mg of phosphorus, and 14mg of sodium. Watercress is high in vitamins A and C.
- **Watermelon:** One cup of diced watermelon provides around 170mg of potassium, 11mg of phosphorus, and 2mg of sodium. Watermelons are refreshing and high in vitamins A and C.
- **White Beans:** One cup of cooked white beans contains approximately 1189mg of potassium, 189mg of phosphorus, and 4mg of sodium. White beans are a great source of fiber and protein.
- **Zucchini:** A half-cup of cooked zucchini provides about 280mg of potassium, 30mg of phosphorus, and 10mg of sodium. Zucchini is a versatile vegetable high in antioxidants and contributes to healthy digestion.

Remember, though these vegetables are considered kidney-friendly due to their lower potassium, phosphorus, and sodium content, individual requirements may vary. Always consult your healthcare provider or dietitian to understand what is best for your specific dietary needs. Regular blood tests are also crucial to monitor the levels of these nutrients in your body.

Incorporating vegetables into a kidney-friendly diet can be both wholesome and enjoyable. It's all about exploring creative cooking techniques and recipes that enhance the natural flavors while adhering to dietary needs.

1. **Roasting:** Roasting vegetables such as bell peppers, carrots, and cauliflower brings out their inherent sweetness. Toss your chopped vegetables in olive oil, sprinkle with herbs and a small amount of sodium-free seasoning, and roast in a preheated oven until tender.

2. **Grilling:** Grilled vegetables like zucchini, eggplant, and mushrooms have a smoky flavor that adds depth to your meals. Slice them, lightly brush them with oil, and grill on each side.

3. **Sautéing:** This technique works well with leafy greens like Swiss chard or spinach. Sauté with garlic and a dash of lemon juice for a fresh, flavorful side dish.

4. **Soups and stews:** Soups and stews are an excellent way to incorporate various vegetables. Use low-sodium broth and add a variety of kidney-friendly vegetables such as onions, leeks, celery, and carrots.

5. **Fresh Salads:** Prepare a colorful salad with iceberg lettuce, shredded carrots, and sliced bell peppers. Dress lightly with a homemade vinaigrette from apple cider vinegar, olive oil, and your favorite herbs.

6. **Stir-frying:** Cook sliced bell peppers, mushrooms, and broccoli in a hot pan with a little oil for a quick, nutrient-rich side. Use reduced-sodium soy sauce or a squeeze of fresh lime juice for extra flavor.

Experimenting with herbs and spices for flavor is essential rather than relying on salt. Fresh or dried herbs such as basil, thyme, rosemary, and cilantro and spices like turmeric, cumin, and paprika can elevate the taste of vegetables and make your meals more enjoyable. Always adhere to the guidelines provided by your healthcare provider or dietitian when preparing meals.

5

MEAL PLANNING FOR KIDNEY DISEASE

P roper meal planning is crucial for maintaining a kidney-friendly diet. It involves understanding your individual dietary needs, selecting the right ingredients, and preparing nutritious and delightful meals.

Guidelines for Crafting Balanced Meal Plans

1. **Understand Your Dietary Restrictions:** Everyone with kidney disease has different dietary needs. Your healthcare provider or dietitian can provide specific guidelines on what nutrients you need to limit or increase. A kidney-friendly diet typically limits sodium, potassium, and phosphorus while getting enough high-quality protein and other nutrients.

2. **Plan Your Meals and Snacks:** Planning your meals and snacks for the week can help ensure that you have all the necessary ingredients on hand, and it can also prevent you from relying on less healthy, last-minute options. Include a

variety of kidney-friendly foods, ensuring each meal is balanced and filling.

3. **Portion Control:** Pay attention to portion sizes to avoid consuming too much certain nutrients. Use measuring cups or a food scale to ensure accurate portions.

4. **Include All Food Groups:** Your meal plan should include a variety of foods from all food groups – fruits, vegetables, grains, proteins, and fats. This not only ensures a balanced diet but also helps to make your meals more enjoyable.

5. **Stay Hydrated:** It is essential to drink the right amount of fluids. Your healthcare provider or dietitian should provide specific recommendations based on your needs.

6. **Limit Processed Foods:** Processed foods often contain high levels of sodium, phosphorus, and other additives that can harm individuals with kidney disease. Opt for fresh foods whenever possible.

7. **Experiment with Flavors:** Don't rely on sodium for flavor. Instead, try a variety of herbs, spices, and other flavor-enhancing techniques, such as roasting or grilling.

8. **Monitor Your Nutrient Intake:** Keep track of the nutrients in your meals. There are many nutrition-tracking apps available that can make this task easier.

9. **Regular Check-ups:** Consult your healthcare provider or dietitian to adjust your meal plan. Regular blood tests can help monitor your nutrient levels and determine if your diet needs to be adjusted.

Remember, maintaining a kidney-friendly diet can be challenging, but with careful planning and creativity, it is possible to enjoy various delicious and nutritious meals.

Emphasizing Portion Control, Food Combinations, and Timing in a Kidney-Friendly Diet

Portion control is a cornerstone of a kidney-friendly diet. Understanding and implementing portion control can help manage the intake of nutrients such as potassium, phosphorus, and sodium, which need to be limited if you have kidney disease. Use measuring cups or a food scale to ensure your servings are accurate. Over time, this practice can also help you to gauge correct portion sizes visually.

Food combinations also play a significant role in a balanced, kidney-friendly diet. Pairing different food groups cleverly can ensure you receive a wide range of essential nutrients without exceeding your dietary restrictions. For instance, combining high-protein foods with low-potassium vegetables can help maintain a balanced intake.

The timing of your meals and snacks is another critical factor. Regular, well-spaced meals can prevent sudden spikes or drops in your blood sugar levels, promoting overall kidney health. Plan your meals so that you eat roughly the same times each day. This helps keep your metabolism stable and can also prevent overeating.

Remember, while adhering to these guidelines for a kidney-friendly diet is crucial, always consult with your healthcare provider or dietitian to adjust according to your individual needs.

Sample Meal Plans for Different Stages of Kidney Disease

Early-Stage Kidney Disease Meal Plan

This stage is characterized by minimal to mild loss of kidney function. In this stage, the kidneys are beginning to lose their ability to filter waste products from the blood effectively, but symptoms are usually not apparent. It's often diagnosed through routine blood or urine tests that detect elevated levels of certain waste products. Even though the kidneys can still maintain normal fluid and electrolyte balance at this stage, it's crucial to implement dietary and lifestyle changes to slow the progression of the disease. These can include nutrition modification, increased physical activities, maintaining a healthy weight, and regular check-ups with your healthcare provider.

Meal Plan 1

Breakfast: Whole grain toast with a thin spread of unsalted butter, one boiled egg, and a cup of fresh berries.

- Whole grain toast (1 slice): Potassium - 69mg, Phosphorus - 57mg, Sodium - 147mg
- Unsalted butter (1 tablespoon): Potassium - 3mg, Phosphorus - 3mg, Sodium - 2mg
- Boiled egg (1 medium): Potassium - 63mg, Phosphorus - 86mg, Sodium - 62mg
- Fresh berries (1 cup): Potassium - 114mg, Phosphorus - 18mg, Sodium - 1mg

Lunch: Grilled chicken salad with mixed greens, cucumbers, and a homemade vinaigrette.

- Grilled chicken breast (100g): Potassium - 256mg, Phosphorus - 196mg, Sodium - 74mg
- Mixed greens (1 cup): Potassium - 160mg, Phosphorus - 15mg, Sodium - 28mg
- Cucumbers (1/2 cup): Potassium - 76mg, Phosphorus - 12mg, Sodium - 1mg
- Homemade vinaigrette (2 tablespoons): Potassium - 17mg, Phosphorus - 8mg, Sodium - 120mg

Dinner: Pan-seared salmon with steamed broccoli and a small baked potato.

- Pan-seared salmon (154g): Potassium - 628mg, Phosphorus - 252mg, Sodium - 117mg
- Steamed broccoli (1 cup): Potassium - 230mg, Phosphorus - 60mg, Sodium - 64mg
- Small baked potato: Potassium - 738mg, Phosphorus - 121mg, Sodium - 17mg

Snacks: A small apple or a handful of unsalted almonds.

- Small apple (150g): Potassium - 195mg, Phosphorus - 20mg, Sodium - 2mg
- Unsalted almonds (1 ounce): Potassium - 200mg, Phosphorus - 137mg, Sodium - 0mg

Meal Plan 2

Breakfast: Rolled oats topped with sliced bananas and a drizzle of honey.

- Rolled oats (1 cup cooked): Potassium - 164mg, Phosphorus - 180mg, Sodium - 115mg
- Sliced bananas (1 medium): Potassium - 422mg, Phosphorus - 26mg, Sodium - 1mg
- Honey (1 tablespoon): Potassium - 11mg, Phosphorus - 1mg, Sodium - 1mg

Lunch: Tuna salad with celery, carrots, and a light mayonnaise dressing served on a whole grain wrap.

- Tuna, canned in water (3 ounces drained): Potassium - 201mg, Phosphorus - 187mg, Sodium - 307mg
- Celery (1/2 cup chopped): Potassium - 180mg, Phosphorus - 11mg, Sodium - 81mg
- Carrots (1/2 cup chopped): Potassium - 205mg, Phosphorus - 24mg, Sodium - 45mg

- Light mayonnaise (1 tablespoon): Potassium - 5mg, Phosphorus - 3mg, Sodium - 105mg
- Whole grain wrap (1 medium): Potassium - 210mg, Phosphorus - 95mg, Sodium - 300mg

Dinner: Lean pork loin with green beans and wild rice.

- Lean pork loin (3 ounces): Potassium - 382mg, Phosphorus - 217mg, Sodium - 48mg
- Green beans (1 cup): Potassium - 211mg, Phosphorus - 38mg, Sodium - 7mg
- Wild rice (1 cup cooked): Potassium - 166mg, Phosphorus - 134mg, Sodium - 5mg

Snacks: A cup of unsweetened Greek yogurt or a pear.

- Unsweetened Greek yogurt (1 cup): Potassium - 240mg, Phosphorus - 233mg, Sodium - 85mg
- Pear (1 medium): Potassium - 206mg, Phosphorus - 22mg, Sodium - 2mg

Meal Plan 3

Breakfast: Scrambled eggs with sautéed bell peppers and onions.

- Scrambled eggs (2 medium): Potassium - 126mg, Phosphorus - 172mg, Sodium - 124mg
- Sautéed bell peppers (1/2 cup): Potassium - 117mg, Phosphorus - 19mg, Sodium - 3mg
- Onions (1/4 cup): Potassium - 61mg, Phosphorus - 20mg, Sodium - 1mg

Lunch: Turkey sandwich on whole wheat bread with lettuce and tomato.

- Turkey (3 ounces): Potassium - 252mg, Phosphorus - 196mg, Sodium - 63mg
- Whole wheat bread (2 slices): Potassium - 160mg, Phosphorus - 138mg, Sodium - 294mg
- Lettuce (1 leaf): Potassium - 70mg, Phosphorus - 3mg, Sodium - 3mg
- Tomato (1 slice): Potassium - 80mg, Phosphorus - 5mg, Sodium - 1mg

Dinner: Baked chicken breast with quinoa and steamed zucchini.

- Baked chicken breast (154g): Potassium - 332mg, Phosphorus - 211mg, Sodium - 104mg
- Quinoa (1 cup cooked): Potassium - 318mg, Phosphorus - 281mg, Sodium - 13mg
- Steamed zucchini (1 cup): Potassium - 345mg, Phosphorus - 58mg, Sodium - 16mg

Snacks: A handful of raw carrots or a small peach.

- Raw carrots (1 medium): Potassium - 195mg, Phosphorus - 25mg, Sodium - 42mg
- Small peach (1 medium): Potassium - 230mg, Phosphorus - 20mg, Sodium - 0mg

Meal Plan 4

Breakfast: Whole grain cereal with low-fat milk and a small orange.

- Whole grain cereal (1 cup): Potassium - 70mg, Phosphorus - 95mg, Sodium - 150mg
- Low-fat milk (1 cup): Potassium - 382mg, Phosphorus - 247mg, Sodium - 107mg
- Small orange (1 medium): Potassium - 174mg, Phosphorus - 18mg, Sodium - 0mg

Lunch: Lentil soup with a side salad of spinach, cherry tomatoes, and balsamic vinaigrette.

- Lentil soup (1 cup): Potassium - 365mg, Phosphorus - 180mg, Sodium - 730mg
- Spinach (1 cup): Potassium - 167mg, Phosphorus - 15mg, Sodium - 24mg
- Cherry tomatoes (1/2 cup): Potassium - 180mg, Phosphorus - 15mg, Sodium - 6mg
- Balsamic vinaigrette (2 tablespoons): Potassium - 27mg, Phosphorus - 3mg, Sodium - 280mg

Dinner: Grilled shrimp with brown rice and steamed asparagus.

- Grilled shrimp (100g): Potassium - 185mg, Phosphorus - 153mg, Sodium - 148mg
- Brown rice (1 cup cooked): Potassium - 154mg, Phosphorus - 162mg, Sodium - 10mg
- Steamed asparagus (1 cup): Potassium - 271mg, Phosphorus - 70mg, Sodium - 2mg

Snacks: A small bunch of grapes or a few slices of cantaloupe.

- Grapes (1 small bunch): Potassium - 288mg, Phosphorus - 20mg, Sodium - 3mg
- Cantaloupe (1 cup): Potassium - 427mg, Phosphorus - 22mg, Sodium - 28mg

Meal Plan 5

Breakfast: Whole wheat pancakes topped with fresh blueberries.

- Whole wheat pancakes (2 medium): Potassium - 183mg, Phosphorus - 98mg, Sodium - 431mg

- Fresh blueberries (1/2 cup): Potassium - 57mg, Phosphorus - 9mg, Sodium - 1mg

Lunch: Turkey and Swiss cheese wrap with mustard, lettuce, and tomato.

- Turkey (3 ounces): Potassium - 252mg, Phosphorus - 196mg, Sodium - 63mg
- Swiss cheese (1 slice): Potassium - 22mg, Phosphorus - 106mg, Sodium - 54mg
- Mustard (1 teaspoon): Potassium - 11mg, Phosphorus - 6mg, Sodium - 57mg
- Lettuce (1 leaf): Potassium - 70mg, Phosphorus - 3mg, Sodium - 3mg
- Tomato (1 slice): Potassium - 80mg, Phosphorus - 5mg, Sodium - 1mg

Dinner: Baked cod with a side of mixed vegetables and a small serving of pasta.

- Baked cod (3 ounces): Potassium - 439mg, Phosphorus - 211mg, Sodium - 82mg
- Mixed vegetables (1 cup): Potassium - 177mg, Phosphorus - 59mg, Sodium - 38mg
- Pasta (1 cup cooked): Potassium - 63mg, Phosphorus - 44mg, Sodium - 1mg

Snacks: A slice of melon or a small handful of walnuts.

- Melon (1 slice): Potassium - 170mg, Phosphorus - 15mg, Sodium - 22mg
- Walnuts (1 ounce): Potassium - 125mg, Phosphorus - 98mg, Sodium - 1mg

Meal Plan 6

Breakfast: Fruit smoothie made with low-fat yogurt, strawberries, and bananas.

- Low-fat yogurt (1 cup): Potassium - 380mg, Phosphorus - 385mg, Sodium - 160mg
- Strawberries (1/2 cup): Potassium - 110mg, Phosphorus - 15mg, Sodium - 1mg
- Bananas (1 medium): Potassium - 422mg, Phosphorus - 26mg, Sodium - 1mg

Lunch: Quinoa salad with cherry tomatoes, cucumber, and a lemon vinaigrette.

- Quinoa (1 cup cooked): Potassium - 318mg, Phosphorus - 281mg, Sodium - 13mg
- Cherry tomatoes (1/2 cup): Potassium - 180mg, Phosphorus - 15mg, Sodium - 6mg
- Cucumber (1/2 cup): Potassium - 76mg, Phosphorus - 12mg, Sodium - 1mg
- Lemon vinaigrette (2 tablespoons): Potassium - 8mg, Phosphorus - 1mg, Sodium - 60mg

Dinner: Grilled chicken with a side of sweet potatoes and steamed broccoli.

- Grilled chicken (3 ounces): Potassium - 256mg, Phosphorus - 182mg, Sodium - 69mg
- Sweet potatoes (1 medium): Potassium - 438mg, Phosphorus - 47mg, Sodium - 72mg
- Steamed broccoli (1 cup): Potassium - 288mg, Phosphorus - 60mg, Sodium - 64mg

Snacks: A small apple or a handful of raw almonds.

- Apple (1 small): Potassium - 147mg, Phosphorus - 11mg, Sodium - 1mg
- Raw almonds (1 ounce): Potassium - 200mg, Phosphorus - 137mg, Sodium - 0mg

Meal Plan 7

Breakfast: Scrambled egg whites with whole grain toast and a small orange.

- Egg whites (1 cup, scrambled): Potassium - 457mg, Phosphorus - 52mg, Sodium - 176mg
- Whole grain toast (1 slice): Potassium - 69mg, Phosphorus - 57mg, Sodium - 147mg
- Small orange (1 medium): Potassium - 174mg, Phosphorus - 18mg, Sodium - 0mg

Lunch: Grilled chicken Caesar salad with a light dressing.

- Grilled chicken (3 ounces): Potassium - 256mg, Phosphorus - 182mg, Sodium - 69mg
- Caesar salad (2 cups): Potassium - 287mg, Phosphorus - 101mg, Sodium - 407mg
- Light Caesar dressing (2 tablespoons): Potassium - 8mg, Phosphorus - 4mg, Sodium - 280mg

Dinner: Baked tilapia with quinoa and steamed green beans.

- Baked tilapia (3 ounces): Potassium - 379mg, Phosphorus - 210mg, Sodium - 58mg
- Quinoa (1 cup cooked): Potassium - 318mg, Phosphorus - 281mg, Sodium - 13mg

- Steamed green beans (1 cup): Potassium - 211mg, Phosphorus - 38mg, Sodium - 7mg

Snacks: A small banana or a few slices of fresh pineapple.

- Banana (1 small): Potassium - 362mg, Phosphorus - 22mg, Sodium - 1mg
- Fresh pineapple (1 slice): Potassium - 120mg, Phosphorus - 8mg, Sodium - 1mg

Please note that these values are approximate and can vary based on each food item's specific brand or variety. Always consult your healthcare provider or dietitian for advice tailored to your circumstances.

Meal Plan 8

Breakfast: Oatmeal topped with fresh raspberries and a drizzle of honey.

- Oatmeal (1 cup cooked): Potassium - 164mg, Phosphorus - 180mg, Sodium - 115mg
- Fresh raspberries (1/2 cup): Potassium - 93mg, Phosphorus - 15mg, Sodium - 1mg
- Honey (1 tablespoon): Potassium - 11mg, Phosphorus - 1mg, Sodium - 1mg

Lunch: Turkey and cheese sandwich on whole grain bread with lettuce and tomato.

- Turkey (3 ounces): Potassium - 252mg, Phosphorus - 196mg, Sodium - 63mg
- Cheese (1 slice): Potassium - 28mg, Phosphorus - 112mg, Sodium - 174mg
- Whole grain bread (2 slices): Potassium - 138mg, Phosphorus - 114mg, Sodium - 294mg

- Lettuce (1 leaf): Potassium - 70mg, Phosphorus - 3mg, Sodium - 3mg
- Tomato (1 slice): Potassium - 80mg, Phosphorus - 5mg, Sodium - 1mg

Dinner: Baked salmon with a side of brown rice and steamed vegetables.

- Baked salmon (3 ounces): Potassium - 416mg, Phosphorus - 252mg, Sodium - 50mg
- Brown Rice (1 cup cooked): Potassium - 154mg, Phosphorus - 162mg, Sodium - 10mg
- Steamed vegetables (1 cup): Potassium - 211mg, Phosphorus - 60mg, Sodium - 28mg

Snacks: A small bunch of grapes or a handful of unsalted cashews.

- Grapes (1 small bunch): Potassium - 288mg, Phosphorus - 20mg, Sodium - 3mg
- Unsalted cashews (1 ounce): Potassium - 187mg, Phosphorus - 168mg, Sodium - 12mg

Meal Plan 9

Breakfast: Greek yogurt topped with a handful of granola and sliced strawberries.

- Greek yogurt (1 cup): Potassium - 240mg, Phosphorus - 245mg, Sodium - 95mg
- Granola (1/2 cup): Potassium - 160mg, Phosphorus - 180mg, Sodium - 10mg
- Sliced strawberries (1/2 cup): Potassium - 110mg, Phosphorus - 15mg, Sodium - 1mg

Lunch: A bowl of chicken noodle soup with mixed green salad.

- Chicken noodle soup (1 cup): Potassium - 300mg, Phosphorus - 50mg, Sodium - 110mg
- Mixed green salad (2 cups): Potassium - 300mg, Phosphorus - 40mg, Sodium - 50mg

Dinner: Grilled lean steak with mashed potatoes and steamed spinach.

- Grilled lean steak (3 ounces): Potassium - 310mg, Phosphorus - 210mg, Sodium - 60mg
- Mashed potatoes (1 cup): Potassium - 620mg, Phosphorus - 60mg, Sodium - 70mg
- Steamed spinach (1 cup): Potassium - 420mg, Phosphorus - 40mg, Sodium - 125mg

Snacks: A small apple or a few slices of fresh cantaloupe.

- Apple (1 small): Potassium - 147mg, Phosphorus - 11mg, Sodium - 1mg
- Fresh cantaloupe (1 slice): Potassium - 180mg, Phosphorus - 15mg, Sodium - 20mg

Meal Plan 10

Breakfast: Whole grain toast with natural peanut butter and a small banana.

- Whole grain toast (2 slices): Potassium - 138mg, Phosphorus - 114mg, Sodium - 294mg
- Natural peanut butter (2 tablespoons): Potassium - 208mg, Phosphorus - 107mg, Sodium - 147mg
- Banana (1 small): Potassium - 362mg, Phosphorus - 22mg, Sodium - 1mg

Lunch: Veggie wrap with hummus, cucumber, bell peppers, and spinach on a whole-grain tortilla.

- Hummus (2 tablespoons): Potassium - 50mg, Phosphorus - 60mg, Sodium - 130mg
- Cucumber (3 slices): Potassium - 23mg, Phosphorus - 5mg, Sodium - 1mg
- Bell peppers (1/2 cup, sliced): Potassium - 117mg, Phosphorus - 15mg, Sodium - 3mg
- Spinach (1 cup): Potassium - 167mg, Phosphorus - 15mg, Sodium - 24mg
- Whole grain tortilla (1 medium): Potassium - 99mg, Phosphorus - 97mg, Sodium - 471mg

Dinner: Baked chicken with a side of couscous and sautéed zucchini.

- Baked chicken (3 ounces): Potassium - 256mg, Phosphorus - 182mg, Sodium - 69mg
- Couscous (1 cup, cooked): Potassium - 91mg, Phosphorus - 66mg, Sodium - 8mg
- Sautéed zucchini (1 cup): Potassium - 345mg, Phosphorus - 57mg, Sodium - 16mg

Snacks: A small pear or a handful of unsalted pistachios.

- Pear (1 small): Potassium - 206mg, Phosphorus - 12mg, Sodium - 1mg
- Unsalted pistachios (1 ounce): Potassium - 285mg, Phosphorus - 137mg, Sodium - 0mg

Mid-Stage Kidney Disease Meal Plan

The mid-stage kidney disease, often referred to as moderate chronic kidney disease, is typically characterized by a more noticeable reduction in kidney function. In this stage, the kidneys struggle to filter waste and excess blood fluids efficiently. Symptoms may manifest, including fatigue, changes in urinary patterns, fluid retention, and difficulties in concentration. Regular monitoring by healthcare professionals is critical, with an increased emphasis on dietary restrictions to manage the disease's progression. At this stage, limiting protein intake, controlling blood pressure and blood sugar levels, and reducing sodium, potassium, and phosphorous in the diet becomes paramount.

Meal Plan 1

Breakfast: A bowl of oatmeal topped with a small amount of honey and half a sliced banana.

- Oatmeal (1 cup cooked): Potassium - 164mg, Phosphorus - 180mg, Sodium - 115mg
- Honey (1 tablespoon): Potassium - 11mg, Phosphorus - 1mg, Sodium - 1mg
- Banana (1/2 small): Potassium - 181mg, Phosphorus - 11mg, Sodium - 0.5mg

Lunch: Tuna salad made with low-sodium canned tuna, light mayonnaise, celery, and onions, served on a bed of lettuce.

- Low-sodium canned tuna (3 ounces): Potassium - 200mg, Phosphorus - 200mg, Sodium - 50mg
- Light mayonnaise (1 tablespoon): Potassium - 5mg, Phosphorus - 5mg, Sodium - 105mg
- Celery (1/2 cup): Potassium - 180mg, Phosphorus - 15mg, Sodium - 80mg
- Onions (1/2 cup): Potassium - 146mg, Phosphorus - 23mg, Sodium - 2mg
- Lettuce (1 cup): Potassium - 140mg, Phosphorus - 20mg, Sodium - 5mg

Dinner: Chicken stir-fry with bell peppers, onions, mushrooms, and a low-sodium soy sauce, served with brown rice.

- Chicken (3 ounces): Potassium - 215mg, Phosphorus - 190mg, Sodium - 70mg
- Bell peppers (1/2 cup): Potassium - 117mg, Phosphorus - 15mg, Sodium - 3mg
- Onions (1/2 cup): Potassium - 146mg, Phosphorus - 23mg, Sodium - 2mg
- Mushrooms (1/2 cup): Potassium - 223mg, Phosphorus - 42mg, Sodium - 3mg
- Low-sodium soy sauce (1 tablespoon): Potassium - 10mg, Phosphorus - 8mg, Sodium - 575mg
- Brown Rice (1 cup cooked): Potassium - 154mg, Phosphorus - 162mg, Sodium - 10mg

Snacks: A small peach or a cup of unsweetened yogurt.

- Peach (1 small): Potassium - 285mg, Phosphorus - 20mg, Sodium - 0mg
- Unsweetened yogurt (1 cup): Potassium - 380mg, Phosphorus - 233mg, Sodium - 100mg

Meal Plan 2

Breakfast: Scrambled eggs with grated cheese and a slice of whole-grain toast.

- Scrambled eggs (2 large): Potassium - 122mg, Phosphorus - 186mg, Sodium - 124mg
- Grated cheese (1/4 cup): Potassium - 27mg, Phosphorus - 303mg, Sodium - 176mg
- Whole grain toast (1 slice): Potassium - 69mg, Phosphorus - 57mg, Sodium - 147mg

Lunch: Turkey sandwich with whole grain bread with lettuce, tomato, and mayonnaise.

- Turkey (3 ounces): Potassium - 252mg, Phosphorus - 196mg, Sodium - 63mg
- Lettuce (1 leaf): Potassium - 70mg, Phosphorus - 3mg, Sodium - 3mg
- Tomato (1 slice): Potassium - 80mg, Phosphorus - 5mg, Sodium - 1mg
- Mayonnaise (1 tablespoon): Potassium - 5mg, Phosphorus - 5mg, Sodium - 105mg
- Whole grain bread (2 slices): Potassium - 138mg, Phosphorus - 114mg, Sodium - 294mg

Dinner: Grilled fish with a side of steamed broccoli and wild rice.

- Grilled fish (3 ounces): Potassium - 414mg, Phosphorus - 235mg, Sodium - 58mg
- Steamed broccoli (1 cup): Potassium - 230mg, Phosphorus - 60mg, Sodium - 64mg
- Wild rice (1 cup cooked): Potassium - 166mg, Phosphorus - 134mg, Sodium - 5mg

Snacks: A handful of blueberries or a small orange.

- Blueberries (1/2 cup): Potassium - 57mg, Phosphorus - 9mg, Sodium - 1mg
- Orange (1 small): Potassium - 174mg, Phosphorus - 13mg, Sodium - 1mg

Meal Plan 3

Breakfast: Scrambled egg whites with diced tomatoes and a side of whole wheat toast.

- Egg whites (2 large): Potassium - 108mg, Phosphorus - 5mg, Sodium - 166mg
- Diced tomatoes (1/2 cup): Potassium - 210mg, Phosphorus - 19mg, Sodium - 5mg
- Whole wheat toast (1 slice): Potassium - 69mg, Phosphorus - 57mg, Sodium - 147mg

Lunch: Grilled chicken salad with mixed greens and a light dressing.

- Grilled chicken (3 ounces): Potassium - 256mg, Phosphorus - 182mg, Sodium - 69mg
- Mixed greens (2 cups): Potassium - 300mg, Phosphorus - 40mg, Sodium - 40mg
- Light dressing (2 tablespoons): Potassium - 10mg, Phosphorus - 0mg, Sodium - 260mg

Dinner: Baked cod with a side of quinoa and steamed asparagus.

- Baked cod (3 ounces): Potassium - 439mg, Phosphorus - 211mg, Sodium - 82mg
- Quinoa (1 cup cooked): Potassium - 318mg, Phosphorus - 281mg, Sodium - 13mg
- Steamed asparagus (1 cup): Potassium - 271mg, Phosphorus - 70mg, Sodium - 13mg

Snacks: A small banana or a handful of raw almonds.

- Banana (1 small): Potassium - 362mg, Phosphorus - 22mg, Sodium - 1mg
- Raw almonds (1 ounce): Potassium - 200mg, Phosphorus - 137mg, Sodium - 0mg

Meal Plan 4

Breakfast: Smoothie made with almond milk, spinach, and blueberries.

- Almond milk (1 cup): Potassium - 180mg, Phosphorus - 24mg, Sodium - 160mg
- Spinach (1 cup): Potassium - 167mg, Phosphorus - 15mg, Sodium - 24mg
- Blueberries (1/2 cup): Potassium - 57mg, Phosphorus - 9mg, Sodium - 1mg

Lunch: Turkey wraps with lettuce, tomato, and a light hummus spread.

- Turkey (3 ounces): Potassium - 252mg, Phosphorus - 196mg, Sodium - 63mg
- Lettuce (1 leaf): Potassium - 70mg, Phosphorus - 3mg, Sodium - 3mg
- Tomato (1 slice): Potassium - 80mg, Phosphorus - 5mg, Sodium - 1mg
- Hummus (2 tablespoons): Potassium - 60mg, Phosphorus - 36mg, Sodium - 120mg

Dinner: Meatloaf made with lean ground turkey, served with steamed broccoli and a small baked potato.

- Lean ground turkey (3 ounces): Potassium - 192mg, Phosphorus - 163mg, Sodium - 70mg
- Steamed broccoli (1 cup): Potassium - 230mg, Phosphorus - 60mg, Sodium - 64mg
- Baked potato (Small): Potassium - 738mg, Phosphorus - 44mg, Sodium - 10mg

Snacks: A few slices of melon or an unsalted rice cake.

- Melon (1 cup): Potassium - 430mg, Phosphorus - 15mg, Sodium - 25mg
- Unsalted rice cake (1): Potassium - 35mg, Phosphorus - 15mg, Sodium - 0mg

Meal Plan 5

Breakfast: Whole grain cereal with unsweetened almond milk and a small orange.

- Whole grain cereal (1 cup): Potassium - 170mg, Phosphorus - 100mg, Sodium - 150mg
- Unsweetened almond milk (1 cup): Potassium - 180mg, Phosphorus - 24mg, Sodium - 160mg
- Orange (1 small): Potassium - 174mg, Phosphorus - 13mg, Sodium - 1mg

Lunch: Lentil salad with cucumbers, tomatoes, and a lemon vinaigrette.

- Lentils (1/2 cup cooked): Potassium - 365mg, Phosphorus - 178mg, Sodium - 2mg
- Cucumbers (1/2 cup sliced): Potassium - 76mg, Phosphorus - 12mg, Sodium - 1mg
- Tomatoes (1/2 cup chopped): Potassium - 210mg, Phosphorus - 19mg, Sodium - 5mg
- Lemon vinaigrette (2 tablespoons): Potassium - 8mg, Phosphorus - 0mg, Sodium - 120mg

Dinner: Baked chicken with a side of brown rice and steamed zucchini.

- Baked chicken (3 ounces): Potassium - 220mg, Phosphorus - 173mg, Sodium - 63mg

- Brown Rice (1 cup cooked): Potassium - 154mg, Phosphorus - 162mg, Sodium - 10mg
- Steamed zucchini (1 cup): Potassium - 345mg, Phosphorus - 98mg, Sodium - 16mg

Snacks: A small pear or a handful of unsalted pistachios.

- Pear (1 small): Potassium - 206mg, Phosphorus - 12mg, Sodium - 1mg
- Unsalted pistachios (1 ounce): Potassium - 285mg, Phosphorus - 137mg, Sodium - 0mg

Meal Plan 6

Breakfast: Quinoa porridge topped with a drizzle of honey and a sprinkle of nuts.

- Quinoa porridge (1 cup): Potassium - 318mg, Phosphorus - 281mg, Sodium - 13mg
- Honey (1 tablespoon): Potassium - 11mg, Phosphorus - 1mg, Sodium - 1mg
- Mixed nuts (1 ounce): Potassium - 187mg, Phosphorus - 136mg, Sodium - 3mg

Veggie stir-fry with tofu and a low-sodium soy sauce.

- Mixed vegetables (1 cup): Potassium - 356mg, Phosphorus - 89mg, Sodium - 38mg
- Tofu (3 ounces): Potassium - 144mg, Phosphorus - 138mg, Sodium - 12mg
- Low-sodium soy sauce (1 tablespoon): Potassium - 37mg, Phosphorus - 8mg, Sodium - 533mg

Pan-seared salmon with a side of sweet potatoes and steamed spinach.

- Pan-seared salmon (3 ounces): Potassium - 534mg, Phosphorus - 252mg, Sodium - 50mg
- Sweet potatoes (1 medium): Potassium - 438mg, Phosphorus - 63mg, Sodium - 72mg
- Steamed spinach (1 cup): Potassium - 839mg, Phosphorus - 101mg, Sodium - 125mg

A cup of unsweetened Greek yogurt or a small apple.

- Unsweetened Greek yogurt (1 cup): Potassium - 240mg, Phosphorus - 233mg, Sodium - 85mg
- Apple (1 small): Potassium - 157mg, Phosphorus - 10mg, Sodium - 1mg

Meal Plan 7

Breakfast: Oatmeal topped with fresh raspberries and a sprinkle of flaxseeds.

- Oatmeal (1 cup, cooked): Potassium - 164mg, Phosphorus - 180mg, Sodium - 115mg
- Raspberries (1/2 cup): Potassium - 93mg, Phosphorus - 15mg, Sodium - 1mg
- Flaxseeds (1 tablespoon): Potassium - 57mg, Phosphorus - 45mg, Sodium - 3mg

Lunch: A roast beef sandwich with lettuce and tomato on whole grain bread.

- Roast beef (3 ounces): Potassium - 210mg, Phosphorus - 162mg, Sodium - 60mg
- Lettuce (1 leaf): Potassium - 70mg, Phosphorus - 3mg, Sodium - 3mg
- Tomato (1 slice): Potassium - 80mg, Phosphorus - 5mg, Sodium - 1mg

- Whole grain bread (2 slices): Potassium - 138mg, Phosphorus - 108mg, Sodium - 294mg

Dinner: Grilled shrimp with a side of couscous and steamed vegetables.

- Grilled shrimp (3 ounces): Potassium - 202mg, Phosphorus - 194mg, Sodium - 805mg
- Couscous (1 cup, cooked): Potassium - 91mg, Phosphorus - 66mg, Sodium - 8mg
- Steamed vegetables (1 cup, mixed): Potassium - 356mg, Phosphorus - 89mg, Sodium - 38mg

Snacks: A small banana or a handful of unsalted cashews.

- Banana (1 small): Potassium - 362mg, Phosphorus - 22mg, Sodium - 1mg
- Unsalted cashews (1 ounce): Potassium - 187mg, Phosphorus - 168mg, Sodium - 3mg

Meal Plan 8

Breakfast: Greek yogurt topped with a handful of granola and fresh strawberries.

- Greek yogurt (1 cup): Potassium - 240mg, Phosphorus - 233mg, Sodium - 85mg
- Granola (1/4 cup): Potassium - 136mg, Phosphorus - 78mg, Sodium - 93mg
- Strawberries (1/2 cup): Potassium - 110mg, Phosphorus - 16mg, Sodium - 1mg

Lunch: Chicken salad with mixed greens and a light dressing.

- Chicken (3 ounces): Potassium - 220mg, Phosphorus - 173mg, Sodium - 63mg
- Mixed greens (2 cups): Potassium - 300mg, Phosphorus - 50mg, Sodium - 28mg
- Light dressing (2 tablespoons): Potassium - 8mg, Phosphorus - 0mg, Sodium - 400mg

Dinner: Baked tilapia with a side of barley and steamed broccoli.

- Baked tilapia (3 ounces): Potassium - 379mg, Phosphorus - 209mg, Sodium - 55mg
- Barley (1 cup): Potassium - 172mg, Phosphorus - 121mg, Sodium - 4mg
- Steamed broccoli (1 cup): Potassium - 230mg, Phosphorus - 60mg, Sodium - 64mg

Snacks: A small bunch of grapes or a few slices of fresh cantaloupe.

- Grapes (1 small bunch): Potassium - 176mg, Phosphorus - 15mg, Sodium - 2mg
- Cantaloupe (1 cup): Potassium - 427mg, Phosphorus - 22mg, Sodium - 24mg

Meal Plan 9

Breakfast: Whole grain pancake topped with a small amount of maple syrup and blueberries.

- Whole grain pancake (1 medium): Potassium - 180mg, Phosphorus - 95mg, Sodium - 350mg
- Maple syrup (1 tablespoon): Potassium - 42mg, Phosphorus - 0mg, Sodium - 2mg
- Blueberries (1/2 cup): Potassium - 57mg, Phosphorus - 9mg, Sodium - 1mg

Lunch: Whole wheat pasta salad with cherry tomatoes, cucumbers, and a light vinaigrette.

- Whole wheat pasta (1 cup, cooked): Potassium - 181mg, Phosphorus - 102mg, Sodium - 4mg
- Cherry tomatoes (1/2 cup): Potassium - 210mg, Phosphorus - 27mg, Sodium - 7mg
- Cucumbers (1/2 cup): Potassium - 76mg, Phosphorus - 12mg, Sodium - 1mg
- Light vinaigrette (2 tablespoons): Potassium - 8mg, Phosphorus - 0mg, Sodium - 260mg

Dinner: Pan-seared turkey breast with mashed sweet potatoes and steamed green beans.

- Pan-seared turkey breast (3 ounces): Potassium - 220mg, Phosphorus - 196mg, Sodium - 55mg
- Mashed sweet potatoes (1/2 cup): Potassium - 214mg, Phosphorus - 36mg, Sodium - 65mg
- Steamed green beans (1 cup): Potassium - 211mg, Phosphorus - 38mg, Sodium - 7mg

Snacks: A small pear or a handful of raw carrots.

- Pear (1 small): Potassium - 206mg, Phosphorus - 12mg, Sodium - 1mg
- Raw carrots (1/2 cup): Potassium - 195mg, Phosphorus - 24mg, Sodium - 45mg

Meal Plan 10

Breakfast: Scrambled eggs with whole grain toast and a small orange.

- Scrambled eggs (2 large): Potassium - 138mg, Phosphorus - 196mg, Sodium - 169mg

- Whole grain toast (1 slice): Potassium - 69mg, Phosphorus - 54mg, Sodium - 147mg
- Orange (1 small): Potassium - 174mg, Phosphorus - 18mg, Sodium - 1mg

Lunch: Quinoa salad with mixed greens, cherry tomatoes, and a lemon vinaigrette.

- Quinoa (1 cup, cooked): Potassium - 318mg, Phosphorus - 281mg, Sodium - 13mg
- Mixed greens (2 cups): Potassium - 300mg, Phosphorus - 50mg, Sodium - 28mg
- Cherry tomatoes (1/2 cup): Potassium - 210mg, Phosphorus - 27mg, Sodium - 7mg
- Lemon vinaigrette (2 tablespoons): Potassium - 8mg, Phosphorus - 0mg, Sodium - 230mg

Dinner: Grilled chicken with a side of brown rice and steamed vegetables.

- Grilled chicken (3 ounces): Potassium - 220mg, Phosphorus - 173mg, Sodium - 63mg
- Brown rice (1/2 cup, cooked): Potassium - 84mg, Phosphorus - 86mg, Sodium - 5mg
- Steamed vegetables (1 cup): Potassium - 356mg, Phosphorus - 89mg, Sodium - 38mg

Snacks: A small apple or a handful of unsalted almonds.

- Apple (1 small): Potassium - 157mg, Phosphorus - 10mg, Sodium - 1mg
- Unsalted almonds (1 ounce): Potassium - 200mg, Phosphorus - 137mg, Sodium - 1mg

Advanced Stage Kidney Disease Meal Plan

In the advanced stage of kidney disease, also known as end-stage renal disease (ESRD), the kidneys have lost nearly all their ability to effectively filter waste from the blood, necessitating dialysis or a kidney transplant. Symptoms are typically quite severe, possibly including nausea, vomiting, shortness of breath, and cognitive impairment. Dietary adjustments remain critical, often with more stringent protein, potassium, and phosphorus restrictions. Fluid intake may also need to be monitored closely. Regular consultation with healthcare providers is crucial to manage symptoms and maintain the best possible quality of life.

Meal Plan 1

Breakfast: Cream of wheat made with water or unsweetened almond milk, topped with a sprinkle of cinnamon and a drizzle of honey.

- Cream of wheat (1 cup, prepared with water): Potassium - 126mg, Phosphorus - 98mg, Sodium - 135mg
- Cinnamon (1 teaspoon): Potassium - 11mg, Phosphorus - 2mg, Sodium - 1mg
- Honey (1 tablespoon): Potassium - 11mg, Phosphorus - 1mg, Sodium - 1mg

Lunch: Sliced turkey breast sandwich on whole grain bread, with lettuce, cucumber, and a light mayonnaise spread.

- Sliced turkey breast (3 ounces): Potassium - 220mg, Phosphorus - 196mg, Sodium - 55mg
- Whole grain bread (2 slices): Potassium - 138mg, Phosphorus - 108mg, Sodium - 294mg
- Lettuce (1 cup): Potassium - 157mg, Phosphorus - 15mg, Sodium - 7mg
- Cucumber (1/2 cup): Potassium - 76mg, Phosphorus - 12mg, Sodium - 1mg

- Light mayonnaise (1 tablespoon): Potassium - 5mg,
  Phosphorus - 3mg, Sodium - 105mg

Dinner: Roasted chicken breast with a small serving of mashed cauliflower and steamed green beans.

- Roasted chicken breast (3 ounces): Potassium - 220mg,
  Phosphorus - 196mg, Sodium - 63mg
- Mashed cauliflower (1/2 cup): Potassium - 150mg, Phosphorus
  - 20mg, Sodium - 15mg
- Steamed green beans (1 cup): Potassium - 211mg, Phosphorus
  - 38mg, Sodium - 7mg

Snacks: Half a pear or a serving of rice cakes.

- Pear (1/2 small): Potassium - 103mg, Phosphorus - 6mg,
  Sodium - 1mg
- Rice cakes (1 cake): Potassium - 14mg, Phosphorus - 15mg,
  Sodium - 32mg

Meal Plan 2

Breakfast: Unsweetened oatmeal with a sprinkle of cinnamon and a small apple.

- Unsweetened oatmeal (1 cup, cooked): Potassium - 164mg,
  Phosphorus - 180mg, Sodium - 9mg
- Cinnamon (1 teaspoon): Potassium - 11mg, Phosphorus - 2mg,
  Sodium - 1mg
- Apple (1 small): Potassium - 157mg, Phosphorus - 10mg,
  Sodium - 1mg

Lunch: Mixed salad with iceberg lettuce, cucumber, and a light dressing.

- Iceberg lettuce (2 cups): Potassium - 87mg, Phosphorus - 21mg, Sodium - 10mg
- Cucumber (1/2 cup): Potassium - 76mg, Phosphorus - 12mg, Sodium - 1mg
- Light dressing (2 tablespoons): Potassium - 8mg, Phosphorus - 0mg, Sodium - 260mg

Dinner: Grilled white fish with a side of couscous and steamed zucchini.

- Grilled white fish (3 ounces): Potassium - 314mg, Phosphorus - 163mg, Sodium - 58mg
- Couscous (1 cup, cooked): Potassium - 91mg, Phosphorus - 74mg, Sodium - 8mg
- Steamed zucchini (1 cup): Potassium - 345mg, Phosphorus - 78mg, Sodium - 16mg

Snacks: Handful of berries or rice cakes.

- Berries (1/2 cup): Potassium - 55mg, Phosphorus - 14mg, Sodium - 1mg
- Rice cakes (1 cake): Potassium - 14mg, Phosphorus - 15mg, Sodium - 32mg

Meal Plan 3

Breakfast: Egg whites scrambled with a slice of whole grain toast.

- Egg whites scrambled (from 2 large eggs): Potassium - 108mg, Phosphorus - 10mg, Sodium - 110mg
- Whole grain toast (1 slice): Potassium - 69mg, Phosphorus - 54mg, Sodium - 147mg

Lunch: Tuna salad with light mayonnaise, served on a bed of lettuce.

- Tuna (3 ounces, canned in water): Potassium - 187mg, Phosphorus - 184mg, Sodium - 338mg
- Light mayonnaise (1 tablespoon): Potassium - 5mg, Phosphorus - 3mg, Sodium - 105mg
- Lettuce (2 cups): Potassium - 300mg, Phosphorus - 50mg, Sodium - 28mg

Dinner: Sirloin steak with roasted cauliflower and a small baked potato.

- Sirloin steak (3 ounces): Potassium - 318mg, Phosphorus - 210mg, Sodium - 55mg
- Roasted cauliflower (1 cup): Potassium - 176mg, Phosphorus - 40mg, Sodium - 29mg
- Baked potato (Small): Potassium - 738mg, Phosphorus - 121mg, Sodium - 13mg

Snacks: A small bunch of grapes or unsalted rice cakes.

- Grapes (1/2 cup): Potassium - 144mg, Phosphorus - 15mg, Sodium - 2mg
- Unsalted rice cakes (1 cake): Potassium - 14mg, Phosphorus - 15mg, Sodium - 32mg

Meal Plan 4

Breakfast: Whole grain cereal with unsweetened almond milk.

- Whole grain cereal (1 cup): Potassium - 160mg, Phosphorus - 180mg, Sodium - 200mg
- Unsweetened almond milk (1 cup): Potassium - 160mg, Phosphorus - 24mg, Sodium - 180mg

Lunch: Vegetable soup with a side salad dressed in a light vinaigrette.

- Vegetable soup (1 cup): Potassium - 466mg, Phosphorus - 82mg, Sodium - 744mg
- Mixed greens (2 cups): Potassium - 300mg, Phosphorus - 50mg, Sodium - 28mg
- Light vinaigrette (2 tablespoons): Potassium - 8mg, Phosphorus - 0mg, Sodium - 260mg

Dinner: Baked turkey breast with steamed carrots and green beans.

- Baked turkey breast (3 ounces): Potassium - 220mg, Phosphorus - 173mg, Sodium - 63mg
- Steamed carrots (1/2 cup): Potassium - 183mg, Phosphorus - 25mg, Sodium - 45mg
- Green beans (1/2 cup): Potassium - 209mg, Phosphorus - 26mg, Sodium - 6mg

Snacks: A small apple or unsalted popcorn.

- Apple (1 small): Potassium - 157mg, Phosphorus - 10mg, Sodium - 1mg
- Unsalted popcorn (1 cup): Potassium - 26mg, Phosphorus - 31mg, Sodium - 5mg

Meal Plan 5

Breakfast: Quinoa porridge with a sprinkle of nuts and a drizzle of honey.

- Quinoa porridge (1 cup, cooked): Potassium - 318mg, Phosphorus - 281mg, Sodium - 13mg
- Nuts (1 ounce, mixed): Potassium - 200mg, Phosphorus - 136mg, Sodium - 1mg
- Honey (1 tablespoon): Potassium - 11mg, Phosphorus - 1mg, Sodium - 1mg

Lunch: Grilled chicken salad with mixed greens and light dressing.

- Grilled chicken breast (3 ounces): Potassium - 220mg, Phosphorus - 196mg, Sodium - 63mg
- Mixed greens (2 cups): Potassium - 300mg, Phosphorus - 50mg, Sodium - 28mg
- Light dressing (2 tablespoons): Potassium - 8mg, Phosphorus - 0mg, Sodium - 260mg

Dinner: Baked cod with a side of quinoa and steamed asparagus.

- Baked cod (3 ounces): Potassium - 439mg, Phosphorus - 163mg, Sodium - 83mg
- Quinoa (1 cup, cooked): Potassium - 318mg, Phosphorus - 281mg, Sodium - 13mg
- Steamed asparagus (1 cup): Potassium - 271mg, Phosphorus - 70mg, Sodium - 2mg

Snacks: A small banana or a handful of raw almonds.

- Banana (1 small): Potassium - 362mg, Phosphorus - 22mg, Sodium - 1mg
- Raw almonds (1 ounce): Potassium - 200mg, Phosphorus - 136mg, Sodium - 1mg

Meal Plan 6

Breakfast: Smoothie with almond milk, spinach, and frozen strawberries.

- Smoothie with almond milk (1 cup): Potassium - 160mg, Phosphorus - 24mg, Sodium - 180mg
- Spinach (1 cup): Potassium - 167mg, Phosphorus - 15mg, Sodium - 24mg

- Frozen strawberries (1 cup): Potassium - 220mg, Phosphorus - 35mg, Sodium - 3mg

Lunch: Turkey wraps with lettuce, cucumber, and a light hummus spread.

- Turkey wrap with sliced turkey breast (3 ounces): Potassium - 220mg, Phosphorus - 196mg, Sodium - 55mg
- Lettuce (1 cup): Potassium - 157mg, Phosphorus - 15mg, Sodium - 7mg
- Cucumber (1/2 cup): Potassium - 76mg, Phosphorus - 12mg, Sodium - 1mg
- Hummus (1 tablespoon): Potassium - 36mg, Phosphorus - 11mg, Sodium - 49mg

Dinner: Meatloaf made with lean ground turkey, served with steamed broccoli and a small baked sweet potato.

- Meatloaf made with lean ground turkey (3 ounces): Potassium - 239mg, Phosphorus - 196mg, Sodium - 77mg
- Steamed broccoli (1 cup): Potassium - 288mg, Phosphorus - 86mg, Sodium - 64mg
- Baked sweet potato (Small): Potassium - 542mg, Phosphorus - 61mg, Sodium - 41mg

Snacks: A few slices of fresh melon or unsalted rice cakes.

- Fresh melon slices (1 cup): Potassium - 431mg, Phosphorus - 19mg, Sodium - 26mg
- Unsalted rice cakes (1 cake): Potassium - 14mg, Phosphorus - 15mg, Sodium - 32mg

Meal Plan 7

Breakfast: Whole grain toast with scrambled egg whites.

- Whole grain toast (1 slice): Potassium - 69mg, Phosphorus - 54mg, Sodium - 147mg
- Scrambled egg whites (from 2 large eggs): Potassium - 108mg, Phosphorus - 10mg, Sodium - 110mg

Lunch: Lentil salad with cucumbers, tomatoes, and a lemon vinaigrette.

- Lentils (1 cup, cooked): Potassium - 365mg, Phosphorus - 178mg, Sodium - 4mg
- Cucumbers (1/2 cup): Potassium - 76mg, Phosphorus - 12mg, Sodium - 1mg
- Tomatoes (1/2 cup): Potassium - 210mg, Phosphorus - 22mg, Sodium - 5mg
- Lemon Vinaigrette (2 tablespoons): Potassium - 16mg, Phosphorus - 0mg, Sodium - 280mg

Dinner: Grilled salmon with mashed sweet potatoes and steamed spinach.

- Grilled salmon (3 ounces): Potassium - 534mg, Phosphorus - 252mg, Sodium - 50mg
- Mashed sweet potatoes (1 cup): Potassium - 509mg, Phosphorus - 63mg, Sodium - 70mg
- Steamed spinach (1 cup): Potassium - 167mg, Phosphorus - 15mg, Sodium - 24mg

Snacks: A small pear or a handful of unsalted pistachios.

- Pear (1 small): Potassium - 116mg, Phosphorus - 12mg, Sodium - 1mg
- Unsalted pistachios (1 ounce): Potassium - 285mg, Phosphorus - 137mg, Sodium - 1mg

Meal Plan 8

Breakfast: Greek yogurt with a handful of unsalted granola and blueberries.

- Greek yogurt (1 cup): Potassium - 245mg, Phosphorus - 385mg, Sodium - 95mg
- Unsalted granola (1/2 cup): Potassium - 136mg, Phosphorus - 167mg, Sodium - 2mg
- Blueberries (1/2 cup): Potassium - 57mg, Phosphorus - 9mg, Sodium - 1mg

Lunch: Chicken salad with mixed greens, cucumber, and a light dressing.

- Chicken salad (1 cup): Potassium - 339mg, Phosphorus - 229mg, Sodium - 540mg
- Mixed greens (2 cups): Potassium - 300mg, Phosphorus - 50mg, Sodium - 28mg
- Cucumber (1/2 cup): Potassium - 76mg, Phosphorus - 12mg, Sodium - 1mg
- Light dressing (2 tablespoons): Potassium - 8mg, Phosphorus - 0mg, Sodium - 260mg

Dinner: Baked tilapia with a side of barley and steamed broccoli.

- Baked tilapia (3 ounces): Potassium - 379mg, Phosphorus - 204mg, Sodium - 85mg
- Barley (1 cup, cooked): Potassium - 174mg, Phosphorus - 121mg, Sodium - 5mg
- Steamed broccoli (1 cup): Potassium - 288mg, Phosphorus - 86mg, Sodium - 64mg

Snacks: A small orange or a handful of unsalted cashews.

- Orange (1 small): Potassium - 174mg, Phosphorus - 18mg, Sodium - 1mg

- Unsalted cashews (1 ounce): Potassium - 187mg, Phosphorus - 168mg, Sodium - 5mg

Meal Plan 9

Breakfast: Pancake made with whole grain flour topped with a small amount of maple syrup and strawberries.

- Whole grain pancake (1 pancake): Potassium - 180mg, Phosphorus - 95mg, Sodium - 210mg
- Maple syrup (1 tablespoon): Potassium - 42mg, Phosphorus - 0mg, Sodium - 2mg
- Strawberries (1/2 cup): Potassium - 110mg, Phosphorus - 16mg, Sodium - 1mg

Lunch: Whole wheat pasta salad with cherry tomatoes, cucumbers, and a light vinaigrette.

- Whole wheat pasta (1 cup, cooked): Potassium - 180mg, Phosphorus - 126mg, Sodium - 4mg
- Cherry tomatoes (1/2 cup): Potassium - 210mg, Phosphorus - 16mg, Sodium - 7mg
- Cucumbers (1/2 cup): Potassium - 76mg, Phosphorus - 12mg, Sodium - 1mg
- Light vinaigrette (2 tablespoons): Potassium - 8mg, Phosphorus - 0mg, Sodium - 260mg

Dinner: Grilled turkey breast with mashed cauliflower and steamed green beans.

- Grilled turkey breast (3 ounces): Potassium - 220mg, Phosphorus - 196mg, Sodium - 63mg
- Mashed cauliflower (1 cup): Potassium - 176mg, Phosphorus - 40mg, Sodium - 15mg

- Steamed green beans (1/2 cup): Potassium - 209mg, Phosphorus - 26mg, Sodium - 6mg

Snacks: A small apple or a handful of raw carrots.

- Apple (1 small): Potassium - 157mg, Phosphorus - 11mg, Sodium - 1mg
- Raw carrots (1/2 cup): Potassium - 184mg, Phosphorus - 25mg, Sodium - 42mg

Meal Plan 10

Breakfast: Scrambled eggs with whole grain toast and a small banana.

- Scrambled eggs (from 2 large eggs): Potassium - 138mg, Phosphorus - 186mg, Sodium - 124mg
- Whole grain toast (1 slice): Potassium - 69mg, Phosphorus - 54mg, Sodium - 147mg
- Banana (1 small): Potassium - 362mg, Phosphorus - 22mg, Sodium - 1mg

Lunch: Quinoa salad with mixed greens, cherry tomatoes, and a lemon vinaigrette.

- Quinoa (1 cup, cooked): Potassium - 318mg, Phosphorus - 281mg, Sodium - 13mg
- Mixed greens (2 cups): Potassium - 300mg, Phosphorus - 50mg, Sodium - 28mg
- Cherry tomatoes (1/2 cup): Potassium - 210mg, Phosphorus - 16mg, Sodium - 7mg
- Lemon vinaigrette (2 tablespoons): Potassium - 16mg, Phosphorus - 0mg, Sodium - 280mg

Dinner: Baked lean pork with brown rice and steamed vegetables.

- Baked lean pork (3 ounces): Potassium - 382mg, Phosphorus - 195mg, Sodium - 57mg
- Brown rice (1 cup, cooked): Potassium - 154mg, Phosphorus - 162mg, Sodium - 10mg
- Steamed vegetables (1 cup mixed): Potassium - 215mg, Phosphorus - 56mg, Sodium - 15mg

Snacks: A small pear or a handful of unsalted almonds.

- Pear (1 small): Potassium - 116mg, Phosphorus - 12mg, Sodium - 1mg
- Unsalted almonds (1 ounce): Potassium - 200mg, Phosphorus - 136mg, Sodium - 1mg

Please remember, these are just sample meal plans. Your specific dietary needs may differ based on the stage of your kidney disease and any other health conditions you may have. Always consult with your healthcare provider or dietitian when creating a meal plan.

Tailoring Meal Plans for Different Dietary Preferences

It's worth noting that the meal above plans can be tailored to fit different dietary preferences while still adhering to the nutritional requirements particular to kidney health. For instance, vegetarians and vegans can substitute meat-based protein sources with plant-based alternatives like lentils, chickpeas, or tofu, bearing in mind that some of these may have higher phosphorus content and should be consumed in controlled amounts. Whole grains, fruits, and vegetables remain essential components of the diet. Still, the choice of these can vary based on personal preferences, with the caveat that potassium content should be monitored. Wheat-based products can be replaced with gluten-free alternatives like rice, quinoa, or gluten-free bread for those following a gluten-free diet. It is critical to remember that these are just examples, and an individual's dietary needs may differ. Therefore, it's always best to consult with a healthcare provider or dietitian when creating a diet tailored to personal preferences and meeting the needs of advanced kidney disease.

6

COOKING TECHNIQUES FOR KIDNEY-FRIENDLY MEALS

C reating delicious and nutritious meals for kidney health requires more than selecting the right ingredients. How you prepare your food can also impact its nutritional value and overall suitability for a kidney-friendly diet. In this chapter, we will explore cooking techniques that can help you optimize your meals for renal wellness.

6.1. Methods of Reducing Potassium, Phosphorus, and Sodium in Cooking

I. **Leaching** - This technique reduces the potassium content in high-potassium vegetables and some types of fruit. It involves soaking and boiling the produce in water to draw out potassium. Vegetables should be peeled, cut into small pieces, and soaked in warm water for at least two hours. Then, the vegetables should be drained and rinsed before being boiled in fresh water. The water should be discarded after boiling.

2. **Cooking with Herbs and Spices** - Instead of using salt to flavor meals, consider using a variety of herbs and spices. Garlic, onion, black pepper, oregano, and thyme are some examples of salt-free seasonings that can be used in cooking.

3. **Steaming** - This cooking method helps retain the natural flavors of food without adding sodium. It is a healthy way to prepare vegetables, fish, and lean meat.

4. **Grilling or Roasting** - These cooking methods allow excess fat to drip away from the food, which can help decrease the phosphorus content in the protein.

5. **Using Homemade Stock** - Most store-bought stocks or broths are high in sodium. By making your own at home, you can control the amount of sodium that goes into it.

6. **Rinsing Processed foods** - If you use canned vegetables or legumes, rinse them thoroughly before cooking to reduce sodium.

Remember to consult your healthcare provider or dietitian to understand how these techniques can be incorporated into your cooking routine.

When it comes to cooking kidney-friendly meals, there are several strategies you can use to ensure that your dishes are not only delicious but also beneficial for your health.

1. **Limit Sodium:** High sodium intake can strain your kidneys and cause other health issues like high blood pressure. Opt for fresh herbs, spices, and citrus to add flavor to your dishes instead of relying on salt.

2. **Control Protein Intake:** Depending on the stage of your kidney disease, you should limit your protein intake. Opt for lean cuts of meat and consider incorporating more plant-based protein sources like lentils and tofu.

3. **Decrease Potassium and Phosphorus:** These two nutrients must be watched closely in a kidney-friendly diet. Limit foods high in these nutrients and be mindful of portion sizes.

4. **Cook from Scratch:** Cooking from scratch allows you to control what goes into your food. This way, you can ensure you're not inadvertently consuming ingredients high in sodium, phosphorus, or potassium.

5. **Adapt Recipes:** Be bold and adapt recipes to make them more kidney-friendly. Swap out ingredients for lower-potassium or lower-phosphorus alternatives and experiment with different flavors.

Remember, the key is to maintain a balanced diet that aligns with your nutritional needs while allowing you to enjoy a variety of flavors and foods.

6.2. Kidney-Friendly Recipes

Here are some kidney-friendly recipes that you can try at home.

1. Quinoa Salad with Vegetables

Ingredients:

- 1 cup boiled quinoa
- 1 cup chopped cucumber
- 1 cup cherry tomatoes, halved
- 1/2 cup chopped bell pepper
- 1/4 cup chopped red onion
- 1/4 cup olive oil
- 2 tablespoons lemon juice
- Salt (as per your doctor's advice) and pepper to taste

Instructions:

Combine all the vegetables in a large bowl. Whisk together the olive oil, lemon juice, salt, and pepper in a separate bowl. Pour the dressing over the vegetables, add the quinoa, and toss to combine.

Serving Size: 1 cup

- Potassium: Approximately ((318mg from quinoa + 152mg from cucumber + 353mg from cherry tomatoes + 144mg from bell pepper + 56mg from red onion + 30mg from lemon juice) / 4) = 263mg
- Phosphorus: Approximately ((281mg from quinoa + 24mg from cucumber + 43mg from cherry tomatoes + 20mg from bell pepper + 14mg from red onion) / 4) = 95mg
- Sodium: This will vary greatly depending on the amount of salt added. Without adding salt, the sodium content is approximately ((13mg from quinoa + 2mg from cucumber + 9mg from cherry tomatoes + 2mg from bell pepper + 1mg from red onion + 2mg from olive oil + 1mg from lemon juice) / 4) = 7mg. Please note that if you add salt, the sodium content will increase.

2. Chicken Stir-Fry

Ingredients:

- 4 boneless, skinless chicken breasts cut into thin strips
- 2 cups mixed vegetables (like bell peppers, broccoli, and zucchini)
- 2 tablespoons olive oil
- Salt (as per your doctor's advice) and pepper to taste

Instructions:

Heat the olive oil in a large pan. Add the chicken and cook until it is no longer pink in the middle. Remove the chicken from the pan, add the vegetables, and cook until tender. Return the chicken to the pan, season with salt and pepper, and stir to combine.

Serving Size: 1 cup

- Potassium: Approximately ((600mg from chicken + 300mg from bell peppers + 505mg from broccoli + 512mg from zucchini) / 4) = 479mg
- Phosphorus: Approximately ((242mg from chicken + 36mg from bell peppers + 105mg from broccoli + 38mg from zucchini) / 4) = 105mg
- Sodium: This will vary greatly depending on the amount of salt added. Without adding salt, the sodium content is approximately ((104mg from chicken + 4mg from bell peppers + 64mg from broccoli + 16mg from zucchini + 2mg from olive oil) / 4) = 47mg. Please note that if you add salt, the sodium content will increase.

3. Baked Salmon with Dill

Ingredients:

- 4 salmon fillets
- 2 tablespoons olive oil
- 1 tablespoon chopped fresh dill
- Lemon slices
- Salt (as per your doctor's advice) and pepper to taste

Instructions:

Preheat your oven to 375 degrees Fahrenheit. Place the salmon fillets on a baking sheet, drizzle with the olive oil, and season with salt and pepper. Top each fillet with chopped dill and a lemon slice. Bake for 12-15 minutes or until the salmon is cooked through.

Serving Size: 1 fillet

- Potassium: Approximately ((800mg from salmon + 2mg from olive oil + 74mg from dill + 30mg from lemon slice) / 4) = 227mg
- Phosphorus: Approximately ((315mg from salmon + 0mg from olive oil + 3mg from dill) / 4) = 80mg
- Sodium: This will vary greatly depending on the amount of salt added. Without adding salt, the sodium content is approximately ((100mg from salmon + 2mg from olive oil + 61mg from dill + 1mg from lemon slice) / 4) = 41mg. Please note that if you add salt, the sodium content will increase.

4. Vegetable Frittata

Ingredients:

- 4 eggs
- 1 cup mixed vegetables (like bell peppers, onions, and zucchini)
- 1 tablespoon olive oil
- Salt (as per your doctor's advice) and pepper to taste

Instructions:

Preheat your oven to 375 degrees Fahrenheit. In a large oven-safe skillet, heat the olive oil and add the vegetables, cooking until they're tender. In a separate bowl, whisk the eggs with salt and pepper. Pour the eggs over the vegetables in the skillet, then transfer the skillet to the oven. Bake for 8-10 minutes or until the eggs are set.

Serving Size: 1 portion

- Potassium: Approximately ((238mg from eggs + 300mg from bell peppers + 146mg from onions + 512mg from zucchini) / 4) = 299mg

- Phosphorus: Approximately ((191mg from eggs + 36mg from bell peppers + 30mg from onions + 38mg from zucchini) / 4) = 74mg
- Sodium: This will vary greatly depending on the amount of salt added. Without adding salt, the sodium content is approximately ((160mg from eggs + 4mg from bell peppers + 2mg from onions + 16mg from zucchini + 2mg from olive oil) / 4) = 46mg. Please note that if you add salt, the sodium content will increase.

5. Berry Smoothie

Ingredients:

- 1/2 cup fresh or frozen berries (like strawberries, raspberries, or blueberries)
- 1/2 cup unsweetened almond milk
- 1 tablespoon honey

Instructions:

Add all of the ingredients to a blender and blend until smooth. This makes a refreshing, kidney-friendly breakfast or snack.

Serving Size: 1 cup

- Potassium: Approximately ((115mg from mixed berries + 186mg from almond milk + 11mg from honey) / 4) = 78mg
- Phosphorus: Approximately ((18mg from mixed berries + 17mg from almond milk + 1mg from honey) / 4) = 9mg
- Sodium: This will vary greatly depending on the amount of salt added. Without adding salt, the sodium content is approximately ((1mg from mixed berries + 160mg from almond milk + 1mg from honey) / 4) = 41mg. Please note that if you add salt, the sodium content will increase.

6. Roasted Garlic Cauliflower

Ingredients:

- 1 head of cauliflower, cut into florets
- 2 tablespoons olive oil
- 3 cloves of garlic, minced
- Salt (as per your doctor's advice) and pepper to taste

Instructions:

Preheat your oven to 400 degrees Fahrenheit. Toss the cauliflower florets with the olive oil, minced garlic, salt, and pepper. Spread the cauliflower on a baking sheet and roast for 20-25 minutes or until tender and golden.

Serving Size: 1 cup

- Potassium: Approximately ((879mg from cauliflower + 2mg from olive oil + 36mg from garlic) / 4) = 229mg
- Phosphorus: Approximately ((176mg from cauliflower + 0mg from olive oil + 14mg from garlic) / 4) = 48mg
- Sodium: This will vary greatly depending on the amount of salt added. Without adding salt, the sodium content is approximately ((49mg from cauliflower + 2mg from olive oil + 5mg from garlic) / 4) = 14mg. Please note that if you add salt, the sodium content will increase.

7. Brown Rice Pilaf with Vegetables

Ingredients:

- 1 cup brown rice
- 2 cups low-sodium chicken broth
- 1 cup mixed vegetables (like carrots, peas, and bell peppers)
- 1 tablespoon olive oil
- Salt (as per your doctor's advice) and pepper to taste

Instructions:

In a large saucepan, heat the olive oil and add the rice, cooking until it becomes slightly toasted. Add the chicken broth, boil, then reduce to a simmer and cover the pot. After 30 minutes, add the vegetables, stir, then continue cooking until the rice is tender and the broth is absorbed. Season with salt and pepper.

Serving Size: 1 cup

- Potassium: Approximately ((154mg from brown rice + 300mg from low-sodium chicken broth + 410mg from mixed vegetables + 2mg from olive oil) / 4) = 216.5mg
- Phosphorus: Approximately ((162mg from brown rice + 50mg from low-sodium chicken broth + 100mg from mixed vegetables + 0mg from olive oil) / 4) = 78mg
- Sodium: This will vary greatly depending on the amount of salt added. Without adding salt, the sodium content is approximately ((10mg from brown rice + 480mg from low-sodium chicken broth + 50mg from mixed vegetables + 2mg from olive oil) / 4) = 135.5mg. Please note that if you add salt, the sodium content will increase.

8. Grilled Chicken with Lemon and Herbs

Ingredients:

- 4 boneless, skinless chicken breasts
- 1 lemon, juiced
- 2 tablespoons olive oil
- 1 tablespoon mixed fresh herbs (like parsley, thyme, and rosemary)
- Salt (as per your doctor's advice) and pepper to taste

Instructions:

Combine the lemon juice, olive oil, herbs, salt, and pepper in a bowl. Add the chicken breasts, turning to coat them in the marinade. Let them marinate in the refrigerator for at least 1 hour. Preheat your grill, then cook the chicken breasts on each side for 6-7 minutes or until cooked.

Serving Size: 1 chicken breast

- Potassium: Approximately ((330mg from chicken + 149mg from lemon juice + 2mg from olive oil + 37mg from mixed herbs) / 4) = 130mg
- Phosphorus: Approximately ((234mg from chicken + 2mg from lemon juice + 0mg from olive oil + 7mg from mixed herbs) / 4) = 61mg
- Sodium: This will vary greatly depending on the amount of salt added. Without adding salt, the sodium content is approximately ((82mg from chicken + 1mg from lemon juice + 2mg from olive oil + 2mg from mixed herbs) / 4) = 22mg. Please note that if you add salt, the sodium content will increase.

9. Baked Apple with Cinnamon

Ingredients:

1 apple

1 teaspoon cinnamon

1 tablespoon honey

Instructions:

Preheat your oven to 375 degrees Fahrenheit. Core the apple, then place it on a small baking sheet. Sprinkle the cinnamon over the apple, then drizzle with honey. Bake for 30 minutes or until the apple is tender. This makes a tasty, kidney-friendly dessert.

Serving Size: 1 baked apple

- Potassium: Approximately ((195mg from apple + 11mg from cinnamon + 11mg from honey) / 4) = 54mg
- Phosphorus: Approximately ((11mg from apple + 1mg from cinnamon + 1mg from honey) / 4) = 3.25mg
- Sodium: This will vary greatly depending on the amount of salt added. Without adding salt, the sodium content is approximately ((2mg from apple + 1mg from cinnamon + 1mg from honey) / 4) = 1mg. Please note that if you add salt, the sodium content will increase.

10. Spinach and Tomato Pasta

Ingredients:

- 2 cups whole wheat pasta
- 2 cups spinach leaves
- 1 cup cherry tomatoes, halved
- 2 tablespoons olive oil
- Salt (as per your doctor's advice) and pepper to taste

Instructions:

Cook the pasta according to the package instructions. In a large pan, heat the olive oil and add the spinach and tomatoes, sautéing until the spinach is wilted and the tomatoes are soft. Add the cooked pasta to the pan, season with salt and pepper, and toss to combine.

Serving Size: 1 cup

- Potassium: Approximately ((180mg from whole wheat pasta + 335mg from spinach + 180mg from cherry tomatoes + 2mg from olive oil) / 4) = 174.25mg
- Phosphorus: Approximately ((152mg from whole wheat pasta + 14mg from spinach + 16mg from cherry tomatoes + 0mg from olive oil) / 4) = 45.5mg

- Sodium: This will vary greatly depending on the amount of salt added. Without adding salt, the sodium content is approximately ((4mg from whole wheat pasta + 24mg from spinach + 3mg from cherry tomatoes + 2mg from olive oil) / 4) = 8.25mg. Please note that if you add salt, the sodium content will increase.

11. Grilled Zucchini

Ingredients:

- 2 zucchinis, sliced lengthwise
- 1 tablespoon olive oil
- Salt (as per your doctor's advice) and pepper to taste

Instructions:

Preheat your grill. Brush both sides of the zucchini slices with olive oil and season with salt and pepper. Grill the zucchini for 2-3 minutes on each side or until they have nice grill marks.

Serving Size: 1 grilled zucchini slice

- Potassium: Approximately ((270mg from zucchini + 2mg from olive oil) / 4) = 68mg
- Phosphorus: Approximately ((38mg from zucchini + 0mg from olive oil) / 4) = 9.5mg
- Sodium: This will vary greatly depending on the amount of salt added. Without adding salt, the sodium content is approximately ((15mg from zucchini + 2mg from olive oil) / 4) = 4.25mg. Please note that if you add salt, the sodium content will increase.

12. Tilapia with Lemon and Dill

Ingredients:

- 4 tilapia fillets
- 1 lemon, juiced
- 1 tablespoon fresh dill, chopped
- 1 tablespoon olive oil
- Salt (as per your doctor's advice) and pepper to taste

Instructions:

Preheat your oven to 375 degrees Fahrenheit. Place the tilapia fillets on a baking sheet, drizzle with olive oil, and season with salt and pepper. Top each fillet with lemon juice and chopped dill. Bake for 10-12 minutes until the tilapia is cooked through.

Serving Size: 1 tilapia fillet

- Potassium: Approximately ((379mg from tilapia + 149mg from lemon juice + 42mg from fresh dill + 2mg from olive oil) / 4) = 143mg
- Phosphorus: Approximately ((204mg from tilapia + 2mg from lemon juice + 1mg from fresh dill + 0mg from olive oil) / 4) = 51.75mg
- Sodium: This will vary greatly depending on the amount of salt added. Without adding salt, the sodium content is approximately ((56mg from tilapia + 1mg from lemon juice + 1mg from fresh dill + 2mg from olive oil) / 4) = 15mg. Please note that if you add salt, the sodium content will increase.

13. Quinoa Salad with Vegetables

Ingredients:

- 1 cup quinoa
- 2 cups water
- 1 cup mixed vegetables (like cucumber, bell pepper, and cherry tomatoes)
- 2 tablespoons olive oil

- Lemon juice to taste
- Salt (as per your doctor's advice) and pepper to taste

Instructions:

Rinse the quinoa in cold water, then add 2 cups to a saucepan. Bring to a boil, then reduce to a simmer and cover, cooking for 15 minutes or until the quinoa is tender. Allow the quinoa to cool, then mix with the vegetables, olive oil, lemon juice, salt, and pepper.

Serving Size: 1 cup

- Potassium: Approximately ((318mg from quinoa + 167mg from mixed vegetables + 2mg from olive oil) / 4) = 122mg
- Phosphorus: Approximately ((152mg from quinoa + 30mg from mixed vegetables + 0mg from olive oil) / 4) = 46mg
- Sodium: This will vary greatly depending on the amount of salt added. Without adding salt, the sodium content is approximately ((2mg from quinoa + 6mg from mixed vegetables + 2mg from olive oil) / 4) = 2.5mg. Please note that if you add salt, the sodium content will increase.

14. Roasted Brussels Sprouts with Balsamic Glaze

Ingredients:

- 1 pound Brussels sprouts, trimmed and halved
- 2 tablespoons olive oil
- Salt (as per your doctor's advice) and pepper to taste
- 2 tablespoons balsamic glaze

Instructions:

Preheat your oven to 400 degrees Fahrenheit. Toss the Brussels sprouts with olive oil, salt, and pepper, then spread out on a baking sheet. Roast for 20-25 minutes or until tender and caramelized. Drizzle with the balsamic glaze before serving.

Serving Size: 1 cup

- Potassium: Approximately ((494mg from Brussels sprouts + 2mg from olive oil + 14mg from balsamic glaze) / 4) = 128mg
- Phosphorus: Approximately ((69mg from Brussels sprouts + 0mg from olive oil + 0mg from balsamic glaze) / 4) = 17.25mg
- Sodium: This will vary greatly depending on the amount of salt added. Without adding salt, the sodium content is approximately ((23mg from Brussels sprouts + 2mg from olive oil + 4mg from balsamic glaze) / 4) = 7.25mg. Please note that if you add salt, the sodium content will increase.

15. Baked Sweet Potatoes with Cinnamon

Ingredients:

- 2 sweet potatoes
- 1 tablespoon olive oil
- 1 teaspoon cinnamon

Instructions:

Preheat your oven to 375 degrees Fahrenheit. Rinse the sweet potatoes and poke several holes in them with a fork. Rub with the olive oil, then sprinkle with the cinnamon. Bake for 45-50 minutes or until soft and tender.

Serving Size: 1 baked sweet potato

- Potassium: Approximately ((438mg from sweet potato + 2mg from olive oil) / 4) = 110mg
- Phosphorus: Approximately ((47mg from sweet potato + 0mg from olive oil) / 4) = 11.75mg
- Sodium: This will vary greatly depending on the amount of salt added. Without adding salt, the sodium content is approximately ((36mg from sweet potato + 2mg from olive

oil) / 4) = 9.5mg. Please note that if you add salt, the sodium content will increase.

16. Carrot and Ginger Soup

Ingredients:

- 4 carrots, peeled and chopped
- 1 onion, chopped
- 2 tablespoons fresh ginger, grated
- 4 cups low-sodium chicken broth
- Salt (as per your doctor's advice) and pepper to taste

Instructions:

In a large pot, sauté the onions until translucent. Add the carrots, ginger, and chicken broth. Bring to a boil, then reduce the heat and simmer until the carrots are tender. Blend until smooth and season with salt and pepper.

Serving Size: 1 cup

- Potassium: Approximately ((410mg from carrots + 92mg from onion + 34mg from ginger + 70mg from low-sodium chicken broth) / 4) = 151.5mg
- Phosphorus: Approximately ((37mg from carrots + 23mg from onion + 5mg from ginger + 18mg from low-sodium chicken broth) / 4) = 20.75mg
- Sodium: This will vary greatly depending on the amount of salt added. Without adding salt, the sodium content is approximately ((69mg from carrots + 4mg from onion + 1mg from ginger + 152mg from low-sodium chicken broth) / 4) = 56.5mg. Please note that if you add salt, the sodium content will increase.

17. Cucumber and Avocado Salad

Ingredients:

- 2 cucumbers, sliced
- 1 avocado, diced
- Juice of 1 lime
- 2 tablespoons olive oil
- Salt (as per your doctor's advice) and pepper to taste

Instructions:

Combine the cucumbers and avocado in a bowl. Whisk together the lime juice, olive oil, salt, and pepper in a separate bowl. Pour the dressing over the cucumber and avocado, then toss to combine.

Serving Size: 1 cup

- Potassium: Approximately ((76mg from cucumber + 487mg from avocado + 12mg from lime juice + 2mg from olive oil) / 4) = 144.25mg
- Phosphorus: Approximately ((24mg from cucumber + 52mg from avocado + 3mg from lime juice + 0mg from olive oil) / 4) = 19.75mg
- Sodium: This will vary greatly depending on the amount of salt added. Without adding salt, the sodium content is approximately ((2mg from cucumber + 7mg from avocado + 1mg from lime juice + 2mg from olive oil) / 4) = 3mg. Please note that if you add salt, the sodium content will increase.

18. Baked Salmon with Lemon and Dill

Ingredients:

- 4 salmon fillets
- 1 lemon, sliced
- Fresh dill sprigs
- Salt (as per your doctor's advice) and pepper to taste

Instructions:

Preheat your oven to 400 degrees Fahrenheit. Place the salmon fillets on a baking sheet, season with salt and pepper, then top each with a lemon slice and a dill sprig. Bake for 20 minutes or until the salmon is cooked through.

Serving Size: 1 salmon fillet

- Potassium: Approximately ((628mg from salmon + 29mg from lemon + 8mg from dill) / 4) = 166.25mg
- Phosphorus: Approximately ((252mg from salmon + 3mg from lemon + 1mg from dill) / 4) = 64mg
- Sodium: This will vary greatly depending on the amount of salt added. Without adding salt, the sodium content is approximately ((63mg from salmon + 1mg from lemon + 2mg from dill) / 4) = 16.5mg. Please note that if you add salt, the sodium content will increase.

19. Rice Pudding with Almond Milk

Ingredients:

- 1 cup short-grain rice
- 4 cups unsweetened almond milk
- 3 tablespoons honey
- 1 teaspoon vanilla extract

Instructions:

Combine all ingredients in a large saucepan and bring to a simmer. Cook on low for 45 minutes, stirring occasionally, until the rice is tender and the pudding has thickened. Serve warm or chilled.

Serving Size: 1/2 cup

- Potassium: Approximately ((30mg from rice + 179mg from unsweetened almond milk) / 4) = 52.25mg
- Phosphorus: Approximately ((22mg from rice + 8mg from unsweetened almond milk) / 4) = 7.5mg
- Sodium: Approximately ((24mg from rice + 180mg from unsweetened almond milk) / 4) = 51mg.

20. Fresh Berry Parfait

Ingredients:

- 1 cup Greek yogurt
- 1 cup fresh berries (like strawberries, blueberries, or raspberries)
- 1 tablespoon honey

Instructions:

In a glass, layer the Greek yogurt, berries, and honey. Repeat the layers until the glass is full. This makes a kidney-friendly dessert that's also perfect for breakfast.

Serving Size: 1 parfait

- Potassium: Approximately ((240mg from Greek yogurt + 40mg from mixed berries) / 4) = 70mg
- Phosphorus: Approximately ((122mg from Greek yogurt + 12mg from mixed berries) / 4) =33.5mg
- Sodium: This will vary greatly depending on the type of Greek yogurt used. Without adding extra salt, the sodium content is approximately ((80mg from Greek yogurt + 1mg from mixed berries) / 4) =20.25mg. Please note that the sodium content will increase if you use regular yogurt or add salt.

21. Grilled Chicken with Lemon and Herbs

Ingredients:

- 4 chicken breasts
- Juice of 1 lemon
- 2 tablespoons fresh herbs (like rosemary and thyme)
- 1 tablespoon olive oil
- Salt (as per your doctor's advice) and pepper to taste

Instructions:

Preheat your grill. Season the chicken breasts with olive oil, lemon juice, herbs, salt, and pepper. Grill the chicken for 6-7 minutes on each side or until fully cooked. Serve with your choice of vegetables or a side salad.

Serving Size: 1 chicken breast

- Potassium: Approximately ((402mg from chicken + 12mg from lemon juice) / 4) =103.5mg
- Phosphorus: Approximately ((247mg from chicken + 3mg from lemon juice) / 4) =62.5mg
- Sodium: This will vary greatly depending on the amount of salt added. Without adding salt, the sodium content is approximately ((87mg from chicken + 1mg from lemon juice) / 4) =22.5mg. Please note that if you add salt, the sodium content will increase.

22. Roasted Butternut Squash

Ingredients:

- 1 butternut squash, peeled and cubed
- 2 tablespoons olive oil
- Salt (as per your doctor's advice) and pepper to taste

Instructions:

Preheat your oven to 400 degrees Fahrenheit. Toss the butternut squash cubes with olive oil, salt, and pepper. Spread on a baking sheet and roast for 25-30 minutes or until tender and golden. Serve as a side dish or add to salads and grain bowls.

Serving Size: 1/2 cup

- Potassium: Approximately ((322mg from butternut squash + 0mg from olive oil) / 4) =80.5mg
- Phosphorus: Approximately ((62mg from butternut squash + 0mg from olive oil) / 4) =15.5mg
- Sodium: This will vary greatly depending on the amount of salt added. Without adding salt, the sodium content is approximately ((0mg from butternut squash + 2mg from olive oil) / 4) =0.5mg. Please note that if you add salt, the sodium content will increase.

23. Bean Salad with Lime Dressing

Ingredients:

- 1 can low-sodium black beans, drained and rinsed
- 1 cup corn kernels
- 1 red bell pepper, diced
- Juice of 1 lime
- 2 tablespoons olive oil
- Salt (as per your doctor's advice) and pepper to taste

Instructions:

Combine the beans, corn, and bell pepper in a large bowl. Whisk together the lime juice, olive oil, salt, and pepper in a separate bowl. Pour the dressing over the bean mixture and toss to combine. Serve as a side dish or add to tacos and burrito bowls.

Serving Size: 1/2 cup

- Potassium: Approximately ((375mg from black beans + 168mg from corn + 161mg from red bell pepper) / 4) =176.25mg
- Phosphorus: Approximately ((100mg from black beans + 32mg from corn + 17mg from red bell pepper) / 4) =37.25mg
- Sodium: Approximately ((25mg from black beans + 1mg from corn + 2mg from red bell pepper) / 4) =7mg.

24. Vanilla Chia Pudding

Ingredients:

- 1 cup unsweetened almond milk
- 1/4 cup chia seeds
- 1 tablespoon honey
- 1 teaspoon vanilla extract

Instructions:

Combine all ingredients in a bowl. Stir well, then cover and refrigerate overnight. Stir again before serving, and add more almond milk to reach your preferred consistency. Top with fresh berries or nuts, if desired.

Serving Size: 1/2 cup

- Potassium: Approximately ((149mg from almond milk + 60.5mg from chia seeds) / 4) =52.375mg
- Phosphorus: Approximately ((121mg from almond milk + 94.5mg from chia seeds) / 4) =53.125mg
- Sodium: This will vary greatly depending on the type of almond milk used. Without adding extra salt, the sodium content is approximately ((10mg from almond milk + 2mg from chia seeds) / 4) =3mg. Please note that sodium will increase if you use regular milk or add salt.

25. Grilled Asparagus and Garlic

Ingredients:

- 1 bunch of asparagus
- 2 cloves of garlic, minced
- 2 tablespoons olive oil
- Salt (as per your doctor's advice) and pepper to taste

Instructions:

Preheat your grill. Trim the ends of the asparagus, then toss with the olive oil, minced garlic, salt, and pepper. Grill for 5-7 minutes, until tender and slightly charred. Serve as a side dish or add to salads and sandwiches.

Serving Size: 1/2 cup

- Potassium: Approximately ((202mg from asparagus + 0mg from olive oil) / 4) =50.5mg
- Phosphorus: Approximately ((26.5mg from asparagus + 0mg from olive oil) / 4) =6.625mg
- Sodium: This will vary greatly depending on the amount of salt added. Without adding salt, the sodium content is approximately ((3mg from asparagus + 2mg from olive oil) / 4) =1.25mg. Please note that if you add salt, the sodium content will increase.

26. Baked Apples with Cinnamon

Ingredients:

- 4 apples
- 2 teaspoons cinnamon
- 1 tablespoon honey

Instructions:

Preheat your oven to 375 degrees Fahrenheit. Core the apples and place them in a baking dish. Sprinkle with cinnamon and drizzle with honey. Bake for 30-35 minutes or until the apples are tender. Serve with a dollop of Greek yogurt or whipped cream, if desired.

Serving Size: 1 apple

- Potassium: Approximately ((195mg from apples) / 4) =48.75mg
- Phosphorus: Approximately ((8.5mg from apples) / 4) =2.125mg
- Sodium: This will vary greatly depending on the type of apples used. The sodium content is approximately ((1mg from apples) / 4) =0.25mg without adding extra salt. Please note that the sodium content will increase if you add salt or use canned applesauce.

27. Sautéed Zucchini and Tomatoes

Ingredients:

- 2 zucchinis, sliced
- 1 cup cherry tomatoes
- 2 tablespoons olive oil
- Salt (as per your doctor's advice) and pepper to taste

Instructions:

Heat the olive oil in a pan over medium heat. Add the zucchini and tomatoes, then season with salt and pepper. Cook for 5-7 minutes or until the zucchini is tender. Serve as a side dish or add to pasta dishes and omelets.

Serving Size: 1/2 cup

- Potassium: Approximately ((512mg from zucchini + 10.5mg from cherry tomatoes) / 4) =130.375mg

- Phosphorus: Approximately ((42.5mg from zucchini + 17.5mg from cherry tomatoes) / 4) =15.25mg
- Sodium: This will vary greatly depending on the amount of salt added. Without adding salt, the sodium content is approximately ((8mg from zucchini + 1mg from cherry tomatoes) / 4) =2.25mg. Please note that if you add salt, the sodium content will increase.

28. Pear and Walnut Salad

Ingredients:

- 2 pears, sliced
- 1/4 cup walnuts, chopped
- Mixed salad greens
- 2 tablespoons balsamic vinaigrette

Instructions:

Combine the salad greens, sliced pears, and chopped walnuts in a large bowl. Drizzle with the balsamic vinaigrette and toss to combine. Serve as a side dish, or add grilled chicken for a heartier meal.

Serving Size: 1 cup

- Potassium: Approximately ((333mg from pears + 62.5mg from walnuts) / 4) =98.375mg
- Phosphorus: Approximately ((6.5mg from pears + 38.5mg from walnuts) / 4) =11.5mg
- Sodium: This will vary greatly depending on the type of balsamic vinaigrette used. The sodium content is approximately ((2mg from pears + 1mg from walnuts) / 4) =0.75mg without adding extra salt. Please note that the sodium content will increase if you add salt or use a store-bought dressing.

29. Roasted Cauliflower with Turmeric

Ingredients:

- 1 head of cauliflower, cut into florets
- 2 tablespoons olive oil
- 1 teaspoon turmeric
- Salt (as per your doctor's advice) and pepper to taste

Instructions:

Preheat your oven to 400 degrees Fahrenheit. Toss the cauliflower florets with the olive oil, turmeric, salt, and pepper. Spread on a baking sheet and roast for 20-25 minutes or until tender and golden. Serve as a side dish or add to curries and stir-fries.

Serving Size: 1/2 cup

- Potassium: Approximately ((293mg from cauliflower) / 4) =73.25mg
- Phosphorus: Approximately ((21.5mg from cauliflower) / 4) =5.375mg
- Sodium: This will vary greatly depending on the amount of salt added. Without adding salt, the sodium content is approximately ((18mg from cauliflower) / 4) =4.5mg. Please note that the sodium content will increase if you add salt or use pre-seasoned turmeric.

30. Quinoa Salad with Veggies

Ingredients:

- 1 cup cooked quinoa
- 1 cup mixed veggies (like bell peppers and cucumbers), chopped
- 2 tablespoons olive oil
- Juice of 1 lemon

- Salt (as per your doctor's advice) and pepper to taste

Instructions:

In a large bowl, combine the cooked quinoa and chopped veggies. Whisk together the olive oil, lemon juice, salt, and pepper in a separate bowl. Pour the dressing over the quinoa mixture and toss to combine. Serve as a side dish, or add grilled shrimp for added protein.

Serving Size: 1 cup

- Potassium: Approximately ((159mg from quinoa + 100.5mg from mixed veggies) / 4) =64.875mg
- Phosphorus: Approximately ((55.5mg from quinoa + 8.5mg from mixed veggies) / 4) =16.25mg
- Sodium: This will vary greatly depending on the amount of salt added. Without adding salt, the sodium content is approximately ((15mg from quinoa + 5mg from mixed veggies) / 4) =5mg. Please note that if you add salt, the sodium content will increase.

31. Baked Sweet Potato Fries

Ingredients:

- 2 sweet potatoes, peeled and sliced into fries
- 2 tablespoons olive oil
- Salt (as per your doctor's advice) and pepper to taste

Instructions:

Preheat your oven to 425 degrees Fahrenheit. Toss the sweet potato fries with olive oil, salt, and pepper. Arrange in a single layer on a baking sheet and bake for 15 minutes. Flip the fries and bake for 10-15 minutes or until crispy and golden. Serve as a side dish or with your favorite dipping sauce.

Serving Size: 10 fries

- Potassium: Approximately ((450mg from sweet potatoes) / 4) =112.5mg
- Phosphorus: Approximately ((37mg from sweet potatoes) / 4) =9.25mg
- Sodium: This will vary greatly depending on the amount of salt added. Without adding salt, the sodium content is approximately ((30mg from sweet potatoes) / 4) =7.5mg. Please note that the sodium content will increase if you add salt or use store-bought fries.

32. Stuffed Bell Peppers

Ingredients:

- 4 bell peppers, tops cut off and seeds removed
- 1 cup cooked rice
- 1 cup cooked black beans
- 1/2 cup salsa
- Salt (as per your doctor's advice) and pepper to taste

Instructions:

Preheat your oven to 375 degrees Fahrenheit. Combine the cooked rice, black beans, salsa, salt, and pepper in a bowl. Spoon the mixture into the bell peppers. Place the peppers in a baking dish and bake for 30 minutes or until the peppers are tender. Serve as a main dish or with a side salad.

Serving Size: 1 stuffed pepper

- Potassium: Approximately ((195mg from bell peppers + 115mg from cooked rice + 207.5mg from black beans) / 4) =129.375mg

- Phosphorus: Approximately ((10mg from bell peppers + 46.5mg from cooked rice + 23.5mg from black beans) / 4) =20.75mg
- Sodium: This will vary greatly depending on the type of salsa used. Without adding extra salt, the sodium content is approximately ((3mg from bell peppers + 2mg from cooked rice + 22mg from black beans) the sodium content will increase) =6.75mg. Please note that if you add sasodium content will increase.

33. Creamy Banana Smoothie

Ingredients:

- 2 bananas
- 1 cup unsweetened almond milk
- 1 tablespoon honey

Instructions:

Combine all ingredients in a blender. Blend until smooth. Pour into a glass to serve. This makes a kidney-friendly breakfast or snack.

Serving Size: 1 smoothie

- Potassium: Approximately ((422mg from bananas + 65mg from almond milk) / 4) =121.75mg
- Phosphorus: Approximately ((22.5mg from bananas + 15mg from almond milk) / 4) =9.125mg
- Sodium: This will vary greatly depending on the type of almond milk used. Without adding extra salt, the sodium content is approximately ((2mg from bananas + 180mg from almond milk) / 4) =45.5mg. Please note that the sodium content will increase if you add salt or use store-bought almond milk.

34. Avocado Salsa

Ingredients:

- 2 ripe avocados, pitted and diced
- 1 small onion, finely chopped
- 1 jalapeño, seeded and minced
- 1/4 cup fresh cilantro, chopped
- Juice of 1 lime
- Salt (as per your doctor's advice) and pepper to taste

Instructions:

Combine all ingredients in a bowl. Stir gently to combine. Serve immediately with kidney-friendly chips or as a topping for grilled chicken or fish.

Serving Size: 1/4 cup

- Potassium: Approximately ((487.5mg from avocados + 36mg from onion) / 4) =130.125mg
- Phosphorus: Approximately ((35mg from avocados + 11.5mg from onion) / 4) =11.875mg
- Sodium: This will vary greatly depending on the type of chips used. Without adding extra salt, the sodium content is approximately ((5mg from avocados + 3mg from onion) / 4) =2mg. Please note that the sodium content will increase if you add salt or use store-bought chips.

35. Blueberry Almond Oatmeal

Ingredients:

- 1 cup oats
- 2 cups water
- 1/2 cup fresh blueberries
- 2 tablespoons almond slices

- 1 tablespoon honey

Instructions:

In a pot, bring water to a boil. Add oats and reduce heat, simmering for 10-15 minutes. Once oats are cooked, stir in honey and top with blueberries and almond slices. Serve warm as a hearty breakfast.

Serving Size: 1 cup

- Potassium: Approximately ((216mg from oats + 70.5mg from blueberries) / 4) =71.625mg
- Phosphorus: Approximately ((112mg from oats + 7.5mg from blueberries + 82.5mg from almond slices) / 4) =50.5mg
- Sodium: Without adding extra salt, the sodium content is approximately ((3mg from oats + 1mg from blueberries) / 4) =1mg. Please note that the sodium content will increase if you add salt or use store-bought oats.

36. Roasted Garlic and Lemon Broccoli

Ingredients:

- 1 large head of broccoli, cut into florets
- 3 cloves of garlic, minced
- 2 tablespoons olive oil
- Juice of 1 lemon
- Salt (as per your doctor's advice) and pepper to taste

Instructions:

Preheat your oven to 400 degrees Fahrenheit. Toss the broccoli florets with olive oil, minced garlic, lemon juice, salt, and pepper. Arrange in a single layer on a baking sheet and roast for 20-25 minutes or until edges are crispy and golden. Serve as a side dish to your favorite protein.

Serving Size: 1 cup

- Potassium: Approximately ((457.5mg from broccoli) / 4) =114.375mg
- Phosphorus: Approximately ((42mg from broccoli) / 4) =10.5mg
- Sodium: Without adding extra salt, the sodium content is approximately ((45mg from broccoli) / 4) =11.25mg. Please note that if you add salt, the sodium content will increase.

37. Pineapple Mint Smoothie

Ingredients:

- 1 cup fresh pineapple chunks
- 1/2 cup fresh mint leaves
- 1 cup unsweetened almond milk

Instructions:

Combine all ingredients in a blender. Blend until smooth. Pour into a glass and serve immediately. This is a refreshing hyd, hydrating, kidney-friendly recipe.

Serving Size: 1 smoothie

- Potassium: Approximately ((182.5mg from pineapple + 65mg from almond milk) / 4) =61.875mg
- Phosphorus: Approximately ((11.25mg from pineapple + 15mg from almond milk) / 4) =6.5625mg
- Sodium: This will vary greatly depending on the type of almond milk used. Without adding extra salt, the sodium content is approximately ((3mg from pineapple + 180mg from almond milk) / 4) =45.75mg. Please note that the sodium content will increase if you add salt or use store-bought almond milk.

38. Spinach and Tomato Frittata

Ingredients:

- 2 cups of fresh spinach
- 1 large tomato, diced
- 4 eggs
- 2 tablespoons olive oil
- Salt (as per your doctor's advice) and pepper to taste

Instructions:

Preheat your oven to 375 degrees Fahrenheit. In a large oven-safe pan, sauté the spinach and diced tomato in olive oil over medium heat. In a separate bowl, whisk the eggs and season with salt and pepper. Pour the egg mixture over the sautéed vegetables and stir gently. Move the pan to the oven and bake for 12-15 minutes or until the eggs are set. Serve as a nutritious and protein-packed breakfast or lunch option.

Serving Size: 1/4 of the frittata

- Potassium: Approximately ((395mg from spinach + 134mg from tomato) / 4) =132.25mg
- Phosphorus: Approximately ((33.5mg from spinach + 23.25mg from tomato) / 4) =14.4375mg
- Sodium: Without adding extra salt, the sodium content is approximately ((39.5mg from spinach + 8.75mg from tomato) / 4) =12.5625mg. Please note that if you add salt, the sodium content will increase.

39. Cucumber and Dill Salad

Ingredients:

- 2 large cucumbers, sliced
- 2 tablespoons fresh dill, chopped

- 1/4 cup white vinegar
- Salt (as per your doctor's advice) and pepper to taste

Instructions:

Combine the sliced cucumbers, chopped dill, vinegar, salt, and pepper in a large bowl. Mix well to combine and refrigerate for at least 1 hour before serving. This dish is a crisp, refreshing accompaniment to any meal.

Serving Size: 1/2 cup

- Potassium: Approximately ((200mg from cucumbers) / 4) =50mg
- Phosphorus: Approximately ((12.5mg from cucumbers) / 4) =3.125mg
- Sodium: Without adding extra salt, the sodium content is approximately ((13.5mg from cucumbers + 2.75mg from vinegar) / 4) =4.5625mg. Please note that the sodium content will increase if you add salt or use store-bought pickles.

40. Carrot and Ginger Soup

Ingredients:

- 4 large carrots, peeled and chopped
- 1 inch piece of fresh ginger, grated
- 4 cups of vegetable broth
- Salt (as per your doctor's advice) and pepper to taste

Instructions:

Combine the carrots, ginger, and vegetable broth in a large pot. Bring to a boil, then reduce heat and simmer for 20-25 minutes or until carrots are tender. Use an immersion blender or countertop blender to puree the soup until smooth. Season with salt and pepper to taste, then serve hot. This soup is a comforting, flavorful option for those on a kidney-friendly diet.

Serving Size: 1 cup

- Potassium: Approximately ((356mg from carrots) / 4) =89mg
- Phosphorus: Approximately ((32.5mg from carrots) / 4) =8.125mg
- Sodium: Without adding extra salt, the sodium content is approximately ((2300mg from vegetable broth) / 4) =575mg. Please note that the sodium content will increase if you add salt or use store-bought vegetable broth. So, using homemade vegetable broth with low sodium is preferable for a healthier option.

41. Apple Cinnamon Oatmeal

Ingredients:

- 1 cup oats
- 2 cups water
- 1 apple, chopped
- 1 teaspoon cinnamon
- 1 tablespoon honey

Instructions:

In a pot, bring water to a boil. Add oats and reduce heat to simmer, cooking for 10-15 minutes. Once oats are cooked, stir in honey, chopped apple, and cinnamon. Serve hot as a hearty and filling breakfast option.

Serving Size: 1 cup

- Potassium: Approximately ((150mg from oats + 130mg from apple) / 4) =70mg

- Phosphorus: Approximately ((50mg from oats + 10.5mg from apple) / 4) =15.375mg
- Sodium: Without adding extra honey, the sodium content is approximately ((2mg from oats + 1.5mg from apple) / 4) =0.875mg. Please note that the sodium content will increase if you add salt or use store-bought oats. So, it is recommended to use plain rolled oats for a healthier option.

42. Zesty Lemon Quinoa

Ingredients:

- 1 cup quinoa
- 2 cups water
- Juice of 1 lemon
- 2 tablespoons olive oil
- Salt (as per your doctor's advice) and pepper to taste

Instructions:

In a pot, bring water to a boil. Add quinoa and reduce heat to simmer, cooking for 15 minutes or until water is absorbed and quinoa is fluffy. Stir in olive oil, lemon juice, salt, and pepper. Serve as a flavorful and protein-packed side dish.

Serving Size: 1/2 cup

- Potassium: Approximately ((318mg from quinoa) / 4) =79.5mg
- Phosphorus: Approximately ((111mg from quinoa) / 4) =27.75mg
- Sodium: Without adding extra salt, the sodium content is approximately ((7mg from quinoa) / 4) =1the sodium content will increase by .75mg. Please note that if you add salt, orum content will increase.

43. Mango Avocado Smoothie

Ingredients:

- 1 ripe mango, peeled and diced
- 1 ripe avocado, peeled and pitted
- 1 cup unsweetened almond milk

Instructions:

Combine all ingredients in a blender. Blend until smooth. Pour into a glass and serve immediately. This smoothie is a creamy and delicious option for a nutritious breakfast or snack.

Serving Size: 1 cup

- Potassium: Approximately ((300mg from mango + 340mg from avocado) / 4) =160mg
- Phosphorus: Approximately ((12.5mg from mango + 21.5mg from avocado) / 4) =8.5mg
- Sodium: Without adding extra salt, the sodium content is approximately ((9.5mg from mango + 7mg from almond milk) / 4) =4.125mg. Please note that the sodium content will increase if you add salt or use store-bought almond milk.

44. Roasted Brussels Sprouts

Ingredients:

- 1 lb Brussels sprouts, trimmed and halved
- 2 tablespoons olive oil
- Salt (as per your doctor's advice) and pepper to taste

Instructions:

Preheat your oven to 400 degrees Fahrenheit. Toss Brussels sprouts with olive oil, salt, and pepper. Arrange in a single layer on a baking sheet and roast for 20-25 minutes or until golden and crispy. Serve as a tasty and nutritious side dish.

Serving Size: 1/2 cup

- Potassium: Approximately ((270mg from Brussels sprouts) / 4) =67.5mg
- Phosphorus: Approximately ((33mg from Brussels sprouts) / 4) =8.25mg
- Sodium: Without adding extra salt, the sodium content is approximately ((15mg from Brussels sprouts) / 4) =3.75mg. Please note that the sodium content will increase if you add salt or use store-bought Brussels sprouts.

45. Watermelon and Mint Salad

Ingredients:

- 2 cups watermelon, cubed
- 1/4 cup fresh mint leaves, chopped
- Juice of 1 lime

Instructions:

Combine watermelon, mint leaves, and lime juice in a large bowl. Toss gently to combine. Serve immediately as a refreshing, hydrating side dish or snack.

Serving Size: 1 cup

- Potassium: Approximately ((320mg from watermelon) / 4) =80mg
- Phosphorus: Approximately ((14.5mg from watermelon) / 4) =3.625mg
- Sodium: Without adding extra salt, the sodium content is approximately ((2.5mg from watermelon) / 4) =0.625mg. Please note that the sodium content will increase if you add salt or use store-bought watermelon.

46. Strawberry Banana Smoothie

Ingredients:

- 1 cup fresh strawberries
- 1 ripe banana
- 1 cup unsweetened almond milk

Instructions:

Combine all ingredients in a blender. Blend until smooth. Pour into a glass and serve immediately. This refreshing smoothie is packed with essential vitamins and minerals, making it a delightful kidney-friendly treat.

Serving Size: 1 cup

- Potassium: Approximately ((150mg from strawberries + 422mg from banana) / 4) =143mg
- Phosphorus: Approximately ((14.5mg from strawberries + 7.5mg from almond milk) / 4) =6.25mg
- Sodium: Without adding extra salt, the sodium content is approximately ((1mg from strawberries + 7mg from almond milk) / 4) =2.5mg.

47. Roasted Zucchini and Squash

Ingredients:

- 1 zucchini, sliced
- 1 yellow squash, sliced
- 2 tablespoons olive oil
- Salt (as per your doctor's advice) and pepper to taste

Instructions:

Preheat your oven to 400 degrees Fahrenheit. Toss zucchini and squash slices with olive oil, salt, and pepper. Arrange in a single layer on a baking sheet and roast for 15-20 minutes or until tender and lightly browned. This simple, flavorful side dish pairs well with various main courses.

Serving Size: 1/2 cup

- Potassium: Approximately ((280mg from zucchini + 260mg from squash) / 4) =135mg
- Phosphorus: Approximately ((30.5mg from zucchini + 18.5mg from squash) / 4) =12.25mg
- Sodium: Without adding extra salt, the sodium content is approximately ((1.5mg from zucchini + 2.5mg from squash) / 4) =1.25mg.

48. Peach and Almond Yogurt Parfait

Ingredients:

- 1 ripe peach, sliced
- 1 cup unsweetened almond milk yogurt
- 2 tablespoons almond slices

Instructions:

Layer the almond milk yogurt, peach, and almond slices in a glass or jar. Repeat the layers until all ingredients are used. Serve immediately or refrigerate for a ready-to-go breakfast or snack. This parfait offers a delightful combination of textures and flavors, plus it's gentle on the kidneys.

Serving Size: 1 cup

- Potassium: Approximately ((220mg from peach + 224mg from yogurt) / 4) =111mg

- Phosphorus: Approximately ((9.5mg from peach + 21.5mg from almond milk yogurt) / 4) =7.75mg
- Sodium: Without adding extra salt, the sodium content is approximately ((2.5mg from peach + 68mg from almond milk yogurt) / 4) =17.125mg.

49. Quinoa and Vegetable Stuffed Peppers

Ingredients:

- 2 bell peppers, halved and seeds removed
- 1 cup cooked quinoa
- 1 cup mixed vegetables, diced
- 2 tablespoons olive oil
- Salt (as per your doctor's advice) and pepper to taste

Instructions:

Preheat your oven to 375 degrees Fahrenheit. In a pan, sauté the mixed vegetables in olive oil until tender. Combine the sautéed vegetables with the cooked quinoa, then stuff the mixture into the bell pepper halves. Arrange the stuffed peppers in a baking dish and bake for 20-25 minutes or until the peppers are tender. This kidney-friendly recipe is nutritious, filling, and packed with flavor.

Serving Size: 1 stuffed pepper half

- Potassium: Approximately ((135mg from quinoa + 95mg from mixed vegetables) / 4) =57.5mg
- Phosphorus: Approximately ((25.5mg from quinoa + 18.5mg from mixed vegetables) / 4) =11.75mg
- Sodium: Without adding extra salt, the sodium content is approximately ((5.5mg from quinoa + 30mg from mixed vegetables) / 4) =8.125mg.

50. Roasted Beet and Goat Cheese Salad

Ingredients:

- 3 medium beets, peeled and cubed
- 2 tablespoons olive oil
- Salt (as per your doctor's advice) and pepper to taste
- 2 cups mixed salad greens
- 1/4 cup crumbled goat cheese
- 2 tablespoons balsamic vinaigrette

Instructions:

Preheat your oven to 400 degrees Fahrenheit. Toss the beet cubes with olive oil, salt, and pepper. Arrange on a baking sheet and roast for 30-35 minutes or until tender. Allow the beets to cool, then combine them with the mixed salad greens in a large bowl. Sprinkle with crumbled goat cheese and drizzle with balsamic vinaigrette. Toss gently to combine before serving. This salad is a colorful, tangy, and delightful addition to your kidney-friendly meal plan.

Serving Size: 1 cup

- Potassium: Approximately ((218mg from beets + 66mg from mixed salad greens) / 4) =71mg
- Phosphorus: Approximately ((14.5mg from beets + 27.5mg from mixed salad greens) / 4) =10.75mg
- Sodium: Without adding extra salt, the sodium content is approximately (2.5mg from beets + 12.5mg from mixed salad greens) / 4) =3.125mg.

So, there are 50 delicious and kidney-friendly recipes to help you maintain a balanced and nutritious diet. Stay hydrated by drinking plenty of water or other kidney-friendly beverages throughout the day. Consult your doctor or a registered dietitian for personalized dietary recommendations, and always listen to your body's unique needs. With these recipes, you can continue enjoying your meals while caring for your kidneys.

LIKE OUR BOOK? LEAVE A REVIEW!

Enjoyed reading our book? Share your thoughts in writing a review! Scan the QR code to leave your feedback and help others discover the inspiring journey within its pages. Your review matters to us!

CONCLUSION

Adopting a kidney-friendly diet doesn't mean you have to compromise on flavor or variety. It opens up a world of delicious and healthy options that can support your kidney health journey.

As the recipes outlined in this comprehensive book demonstrate, you have a wide range of choices when creating delicious and nutrient-rich meals. From savory chicken dishes seasoned with flavorful herbs and spices to refreshing berry smoothies bursting with antioxidants, there are countless ways to nourish your body while enjoying every bite.

By making informed choices about your diet, you can take proactive steps toward maintaining and improving your kidney health. But it's not just about the nutrients you consume; it's also about embracing a healthier lifestyle and truly savoring your food.

To further support your kidney health goals, consider contacting nutritionists specializing in renal health. They can provide personalized guidance and recommendations tailored to your unique needs. Additionally, joining support groups in your local community or online can connect you with others on a similar journey, allowing you to share experiences, learn from each other, and find encouragement.

Remember, this journey can be taken one meal at a time. With every kidney-friendly dish you prepare, you're contributing to your overall health and wellness and cultivating a deeper appreciation for the power of food. Stay committed, stay informed, and most importantly, enjoy nourishing your body and embracing a kidney-friendly lifestyle.

Made in the USA
Las Vegas, NV
09 March 2024

86952649R00194